ORAL AND MAXILLOFACIAL SURGERY
An Illustrated Guide for Dental Students and Allied Dental Professionals

Nabeela Ahmed
Rhea Chouhan
Robert Isaac
Arpan S. Tahim
Karl F.B. Payne
Alexander M.C. Goodson
Peter A. Brennan

Published in 2024 by Libri Publishing

Copyright © Nabeela Ahmed, Rhea Chouhan, Robert Isaac, Arpan S. Tahim, Karl F.B. Payne, Alexander M.C. Goodson and Peter A. Brennan

The right of Nabeela Ahmed, Rhea Chouhan, Robert Isaac, Arpan S. Tahim, Karl F.B. Payne, Alexander M.C. Goodson and Peter A. Brennan to be identified as the authors of this work has been asserted in accordance with the Copyright, Designs and Patents Act, 1988.

ISBN 978-1-911450-87-0 paperback
ISBN 978-1-911450-92-4 hardback

All rights reserved. No part of this publication may be reproduced, stored in any retrieval system or transmitted in any form or by any means, electronic, mechanical, photocopying, recording or otherwise, without the prior written permission of the copyright holder for which application should be addressed in the first instance to the publishers. No liability shall be attached to the author, the copyright holder or the publishers for loss or damage of any nature suffered as a result of reliance on the reproduction of any of the contents of this publication or any errors or omissions in its contents.

A CIP catalogue record for this book is available from The British Library

Cover and Design by Carnegie Book Production

Libri Publishing
Brunel House
Volunteer Way
Faringdon
Oxfordshire
SN7 7YR

Tel: +44 (0)845 873 3837

www.libripublishing.co.uk

PREFACE

Oral and Maxillofacial Surgery (OMFS) is the exciting specialty combining dentistry with medicine and surgery leading to a uniquely specialised and rewarding career which combines this knowledge with the ability to change and improve patients' faces, whether suffering pathology such as oral and pharyngeal cancers, improving dentofacial disproportion, treating children with congenital abnormalities such as cleft and craniofacial syndromes, TMJ and salivary gland pathology or performing facial aesthetic procedures.

Enhancing a smile can be very rewarding in dentistry. The face is our way of recognising who we are in the mirror and how we portray ourselves to others and any change has significant psychological impact and affects our confidence and success in life. The surgeon with an ability to change a face carries thus significant responsibility, but equally achieves greater professional satisfaction when a job is done well and a patient's quality of life is improved.

Most dental students have some exposure to OMFS via Oral Surgery and for those fortunate enough to spend some time with an OMFS team, many are inspired to go on to complete a shortened medical degree and pursue specialty training. OMFS surgeons work closely with allied surgical specialties such as neurosurgeons, ENT, Plastics and Ophthalmology colleagues but also the dental specialities in multidisciplinary teams with orthodontists, prosthodontists and periodontists and the scope of work includes the full remit of Oral Surgery.

The British Association of Oral and Maxillofacial Surgeons (BAOMS) has funded this book to widen awareness of what OMFS surgeons do and to give dental students and allied dental health professionals background knowledge on the scope of OMFS with practical examples of what we do. For the reader, it will give you an idea of emergency and urgent conditions and the likely options for provision of care for your patients when you refer them to us. I hope the book goes further and inspires you to touch base with your local OMFS unit or our dedicated colleagues at BAOMS via our website so we can support your career aspirations if you wish to learn more about OMFS.

Miss Daljit K Dhariwal
62nd President BAOMS

ABOUT THE AUTHORS

Nabeela Ahmed
BDS, MFDS, MBChB, FRCS (OMFS), MMedSci (Med Ed)

Nabeela is a Consultant maxillofacial surgeon based at the Queens Medical Centre in Nottingham. She completed her registrar training across the London and Trent deaneries, and then undertook a 2 year post CCT fellowship in Australia and New Zealand with a trauma and skin cancer interest. Her current clinical practice is facial deformity, both acquired and post traumatic.

She has an active interest in medical education and has authored several textbook chapters in OMFS. She is also an elected fellow on BAOMS council.

Rhea Chouhan
BDS, MFDS, MBChB

Rhea is a dual qualified clinical fellow in Oral and Maxillofacial Surgery (OMFS), currently working in London. She has previously held elected positions as Chair of the Junior Trainees Group of The British Association of Oral and Maxillofacial Surgeons (BAOMS) and Junior Trainees & Members' Representative on BAOMS Council.

Having worked with BAOMS for a number of years, she is passionate about improving access and exposure to OMFS to both medical and dental undergraduates and in retaining current junior trainees by increasing learning and training opportunities. She has authored several papers in OMFS and collaborated with others to create a national mentorship scheme and hopes to continue supporting such projects in future during her training

Robert Isaac
BDS (Hons), MBBCH (Hons), FRCS (OMFS)

Robert has recently been appointed a Consultant in Oral and Maxillofacial surgery (OMFS) in Queen Alexandra Hospital, Portsmouth. He completed both his dental and medical degrees in Cardiff University before being appointed as 'run through' OMFS trainee in the Wessex Deanery.

He has written chapters in the 50 Landmark Papers in OMFS and Bailey and Love Essential Operations in OMFS and has become a reviewer for the British Journal of Oral and Maxillofacial Surgery. He has a particular aspiration to increase exposure to OMFS to both dental and medical undergraduates and holds an active interest in recruitment and retention within the specialty.

Arpan S. Tahim
MBBS, BSc (Hons), BDS, MRCS, MEd, PhD

Arpan is an honorary clinical lecturer at UCL medical school. He completed his PhD at the UCL Institute of Education. He has authored books, chapters and research articles focused on academic and clinical aspects of Medical Education and has set up numerous novel and successful educational interventions. His special interest lies in healthcare-related workplace learning and assessment.

Karl F.B. Payne
BMedSci, BMBS, BDS, FRCS, PhD

Karl is a Specialist Registrar in Oral and Maxillofacial surgery (OMFS) in the West Midlands Deanery, and NIHR Clinical Lecturer at the University of Birmingham. He completed his medical training in Nottingham and Dental training in London. As an academic surgeon, Karl's primary interests are using a blood test to detect DNA mutations from head and neck cancers. Karl has written several chapters and books in OMFS, raising awareness of the specialty at a national and international level.

Alexander M.C. Goodson
BSc (Hons), MBBS, BDS, FRCS (OMFS), DOHNS, PhD

Alex works as a Consultant maxillofacial surgeon at Queen Alexandra Hospital, Portsmouth and is an elected fellow on the BAOMS council. Having completed his specialty training in South Wales and a post-CCT Head and Neck fellowship in Birmingham, his subspecialty interests lie in head & neck oncology, microvascular reconstruction, salivary gland disease and facial nerve injury. He also has an active interest in facial aesthetic surgery and full-mouth dental implant rehabilitation.

He has a complementary clinical research interest in the continuing development of reverse planning and additively manufactured (customised 3D-printed) CMF implants for complex reconstructions with a focus on improving surgical efficiency and quality-of-life outcomes. He has taken an active role in raising the awareness of the specialty, having authored texts for primary care practitioners, as well as regularly teaching for the Midlands and East Deaneries and authoring texts for grass-roots trainees.

Peter A. Brennan

MB BS, BDS, MD, PhD, FRCS (Eng), FRCSI, Hon FRCS, FFST (Ed), FDSRCS

Professor Peter Brennan is a Consultant in Oral and Maxillofacial Surgery (OMFS) at Portsmouth, UK. He has a personal chair in recognition of his education and research profile.

Peter has over 830 publications with more than 80 on human factors (HF) and patient safety. He was awarded a PhD in HF in 2019 and as a trainee, completed an MD thesis on oral cancer biology. He is lead editor of several specialty surgical textbooks including the renowned Gray's Surgical Anatomy, the two volume Maxillofacial Surgery, Oxford Handbook of OMFS and the newly published Bailey and Love's Essential Operations in OMFS.

In 2022, Peter won the coveted Silver Scalpel Award for outstanding commitment to training across all 10 surgical specialties and was awarded an Honorary Fellowship of the Royal College of Surgeons for his achievements in wider surgery. His extensive HF work has helped changed practice, improve team working and patient safety around the world.

Peter is committed to training, supporting and empowering the future generation across wider healthcare.

CONTENTS

CHAPTER 1: THE BASICS 1
1.1 INTRODUCTION 1
1.2 EXAMINING THE FACE AND MOUTH 2
1.3 SOME IMPORTANT INVESTIGATIONS 2
1.4 THE TRAUMA PATIENT 3

CHAPTER 2: THE MOUTH 13
2.1 ANATOMY 13
2.2 ULCERS AND PATCHES IN THE MOUTH 14
    2.2.1 SUSPICIOUS ULCERS 16
    2.2.2 BENIGN ORAL ULCERATION 16
    2.2.3 RECURRENT ULCERATION 17
    2.2.4 ERYTHEMA MULTIFORME 17
    2.2.5 PATCHES 18
2.3 LUMPS AND SWELLINGS IN THE MOUTH 24
2.4 ORAL CANCER 28
2.5 DENTOALVEOLAR SURGERY 34
2.6 CLEFT LIP AND PALATE 38
2.7 DENTAL TRAUMA 41

CHAPTER 3: THE JAWS 43
3.1 ANATOMY AND EMBRYOLOGY 43
3.2 FRACTURES OF THE MANDIBLE AND MIDFACE 43
    3.2.1 MANDIBULAR FRACTURES 43
    3.2.2 MIDFACE FRACTURES 48
3.3 JAW DEFORMITY 53
    3.3.1 ASSESSMENT 54
    3.3.2 EXAMINATION 54
    3.3.3 TREATMENT 56
    3.3.4 DISTRACTION OSTEOGENESIS 58
3.4 THE TEMPOROMANDIBULAR JOINT (TMJ) 58

      3.4.1 ANATOMY   58
      3.4.2 EXAMINING THE TMJ   59
      3.4.3 TEMPOROMANDIBULAR JOINT DISORDER (TMJD)   59
      3.4.4 TMJ DISLOCATION   62
      3.4.5 MECHANICAL OBSTRUCTION OF THE TMJ   63

3.5 CYSTS OF THE JAW   64
      3.5.1 RADICULAR CYSTS   65
      3.5.2 DENTIGEROUS CYSTS   65
      3.5.3 ODONTOGENIC KERATOCYST   66
      3.5.4 AMELOBLASTOMA   68
      3.5.5 METASTATIC DISEASE   68

3.6 MEDICATION-RELATED OSTEONECROSIS OF THE JAWS (MRONJ)   68

3.7 OSTEORADIONECROSIS (ORN) OF THE JAWS   69

CHAPTER 4: SALIVARY GLANDS, THE FACIAL NERVE AND FACIAL PAIN   71

4.1 ANATOMY   71

4.2 SALIVARY GLAND PATHOLOGY   72
      4.2.1 SALIVARY TUMOURS   73
      4.2.2 OBSTRUCTIVE SALIVARY GLAND DISEASE   75
      4.2.3 SALIVARY GLAND TRAUMA   77

4.3 FACIAL PAIN   77
      4.3.1 TEMPOROMANDIBULAR DISORDER   78
      4.3.2 TRIGEMINAL NEURALGIA   78
      4.3.3 ATYPICAL FACIAL PAIN AND BURNING MOUTH SYNDROME   79
      4.3.4 POST-HERPETIC NEURALGIA   80

4.4 FACIAL PALSY   80

CHAPTER 5: SOFT TISSUES AND THE NECK   83

5.1 FACIAL LACERATIONS AND NECK WOUNDS   83
      5.1.1 SIMPLE SOFT-TISSUE LACERATIONS/WOUNDS   83
      5.1.2 DEEP SOFT-TISSUE INJURIES   84
      5.1.3 BITES   88

5.2 NECK LUMPS	88
5.2.1 INFLAMMATORY INCLUDING TISSUE SPACE INFECTIONS	89
5.2.2 CONGENITAL	91
5.2.3 NEOPLASTIC	95
CHAPTER 6: FRONTAL BONE, CRANIUM AND ORBITS	**101**
6.1 INTRODUCTION	101
6.2 ANATOMY	101
6.2.1 SURGICAL ACCESS	102
6.3 TRAUMATIC INJURIES TO THE FRONTAL BONE	104
6.4 ORBITAL FRACTURES	105
6.5 ORBITAL COMPARTMENT SYNDROME	108
6.6 CRANIOFACIAL SURGERY	109
6.7 SKIN CANCERS OF THE SCALP AND FOREHEAD	110
CHAPTER 7: NOSE AND SINUSES	**115**
7.1 INTRODUCTION	115
7.2 ANATOMY	115
7.3 FRACTURES	116
7.4 BLEEDING	122
7.5 DENTAL PATHOLOGY	122
7.6 SKIN CANCERS ON THE NOSE AND CHEEK	123
CHAPTER 8: SKIN PATHOLOGY AND AESTHETIC SURGERY	**127**
8.1 SKIN CANCER	127
8.1.1 MALIGNANT MELANOMA	127
8.2 NON-MELANOMA SKIN CANCER (NMSC)	127
8.2.1 BASAL CELL CARCINOMA (BCC)	131
8.2.2 SQUAMOUS CELL CARCINOMA (SCC)	132
8.3 BENIGN SKIN TUMOURS	136
8.3.1 KERATOACANTHOMA	136
8.3.2 LIPOMA	136
8.4 AESTHETIC SKIN SURGERY	137

CHAPTER 9: ORAL AND MAXILLOFACIAL SURGERY – CAREER AND RESEARCH OPPORTUNITIES 141
9.1 BACKGROUND 141
9.2 BRITISH ASSOCIATION OF ORAL AND MAXILLOFACIAL SURGEONS (BAOMS) 142
9.3 CAREER PATHWAYS 142
9.4 RESEARCH 143

CHAPTER 1: THE BASICS

1.1 INTRODUCTION

Oral and maxillofacial surgery (OMFS) originally developed during the middle of the twentieth century when dental surgeons began to apply their knowledge of the oral cavity and its surrounding tissues to treat military personnel who had sustained potentially devastating facial injuries during various conflicts, including the Second World War.

Since then, the remit of the speciality and the range of various pathologies within it have become increasingly diverse. As cases in the speciality became more complex, it was clear that in addition to a detailed knowledge of the oral cavity and facial skeleton, a firm grounding in the principles of both medicine and surgery was required to best manage these patients. So, in the late 1980s dual qualification in both dentistry and medicine became mandatory.

As dental students, you will be familiar with oral and maxillofacial surgery, as you will have exams in this speciality and, depending on where you train, may even do clinical blocks away from your base hospital to gain an insight into the work of OMFS surgeons. These placements may be the first time you are exposed to the speciality and become interested in finding out more about it, or even consider it as a potential career. Like many other surgical specialities, OMFS shares a tremendous amount in common with the other disciplines across both medicine and surgery. We will showcase the diversity of the speciality with this book by introducing you to OMFS and highlighting the overlap it shares with other specialities. We will take you through the different regions of the face and the different pathologies that patients present with, and introduce ways that OMFS can manage them. While it is by no means exhaustive in its scope and it cannot include all the pathology encountered in this complex anatomical region, we hope this book will inspire you to find out more about the problems that patients can develop in this region of the body.

The impact that disease and treatment in this area can have on patients and their families cannot be underestimated, as it is difficult to conceal the face from the outside world. We hope that the information and knowledge in this book will be useful for all students, whatever speciality or branch of dentistry you decide to pursue – whether that be in general dental practice or one of the many dental sub-specialities including oral-surgery/orthodontics/paediatrics/special-care dentistry, oral pathology, medicine or radiology. Or even, perhaps, OMFS itself.

Please do let us know if you think we should have included other topics too. The purpose of this book is to educate and support the knowledge of those looking after patients daily, and even to inspire some of you considering becoming OMFS surgeons to do so.

1.2 EXAMINING THE FACE AND MOUTH

As with all dental and medical presentations, the cornerstone of management of oral and maxillofacial pathology lies in obtaining a thorough history and examination. One of the challenges to examining the head and neck region is the need for a flexible approach. Your examination is often tailored to the situation, or the information you have picked up from your patient during the history. Similarly, how you examine a trauma patient might appear very different to how you examine a patient with a parotid swelling. However, the following framework should act as a foundation of general principles that you can adapt as you gain more experience.

Many clinical examinations begin by stressing the importance of noting any abnormalities affecting the head and neck. Building on that, we shall take you through a simple examination of the facial skeleton, the dental hard tissues, the oral soft tissues and the neck.

Facial Examination

Simply observing the face at rest allows you to assess for facial asymmetry arising from, for example, facial swellings or muscle weakness. You can make a note of any lesions, bruising or lacerations. It is also useful to see how the jaw opens and closes – which reveals important information about the muscles of mastication and the temporomandibular joint (TMJ) itself. For example,

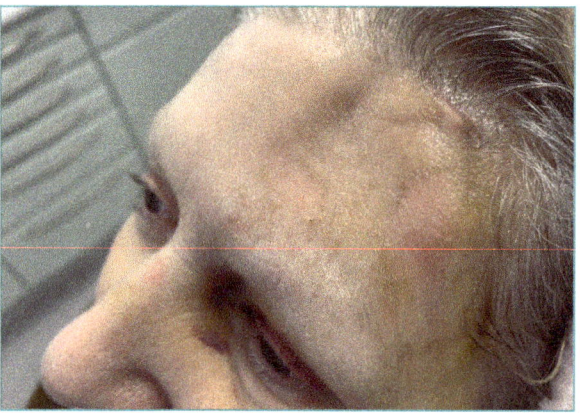

Figure 1.1: Simply examining the patient at rest can help identify obvious deformity. This patient presented with an obvious depressed left frontal bone structure. Picture courtesy of Lieutenant Colonel Johno Breeze

patients might show painful or restricted mouth opening, or even deviation of the jaw to one side as they open.

You can palpate the prominences of the bony skeleton – the orbital rims, the nasal bones, the cheeks (zygoma), the temporomandibular joints (TMJ) (where you can feel crepitus in an abnormal jaw joint) and the mandible itself. As you feel, you want to note if the area is tender, or if there is an underlying bony step that might suggest a facial bone fracture. Sometimes useful information is gained by feeling the bones inside the mouth. For example, midface fractures can be detected by simply grasping the maxilla on either side of the upper teeth and feeling if it is mobile (with your second hand stabilising the frontal bone). As part of the palpation process, remember to check the three divisions of the trigeminal nerve (sensation to the upper, middle and lower parts of the face, and motor supply to the masticatory muscles).

In the trauma situation, it is also useful to screen the eye – often by checking its gross appearance, gross vision, symmetry with the other eye, pupillary response and the range of eye movements. If you do this routinely, any abnormality will be easily picked up.

Intra-oral Examination

Generally, the oral cavity can be examined without any specialist equipment, but it is imperative to have good lighting, and useful to have either a wooden tongue spatula or a dental mirror to hand.

An adult with a full dentition can normally have up to 32 teeth – occasionally more with supernumerary teeth. The tooth-bearing areas are divided into the four quadrants, each containing from the midline outwards: a central incisor, lateral incisor, a canine, two premolar teeth and three molar teeth. The last of these molar teeth are called 'wisdom teeth', but can be absent in some patients. Depending on the nature of the presenting complaint, important things to assess in a patient's teeth are:

a) Any significant dental decay (or caries) – often in the form of physical defects on the teeth or brown discolouration.
b) The presence of composite (usually white) or amalgam fillings and crowns.
c) Any mobility of the teeth, which can be done by simple palpation.
d) Any tenderness to percussion (often done by tapping the top of the tooth with an instrument; if this is painful, it often indicates inflammatory pathology at the tip of the tooth root).
e) Any discharging sinuses on the gums, which are a sign of chronic dental infection.

4   ORAL AND MAXILLOFACIAL SURGERY

---

f) How a patient's teeth bite together (also called their '*dental occlusion*') as they dynamically open and close their jaw. As an example, patients with mandibular fractures often report a change in their bite, as the continuity of their dental arch is disrupted. Often you will see a gap between their teeth, or a step in their occlusion. This evaluation of the occlusion is also very relevant when considering whether patients have an underlying developmental skeletal discrepancy and may require orthodontics with orthognathic surgical input (we'll discuss this later, in Chapter 3).

g) Any absent teeth – and are they accounted for (especially in the trauma situation). For example, a tooth may have been avulsed; could it have been inhaled? Does the patient require a chest x-ray for evaluation?

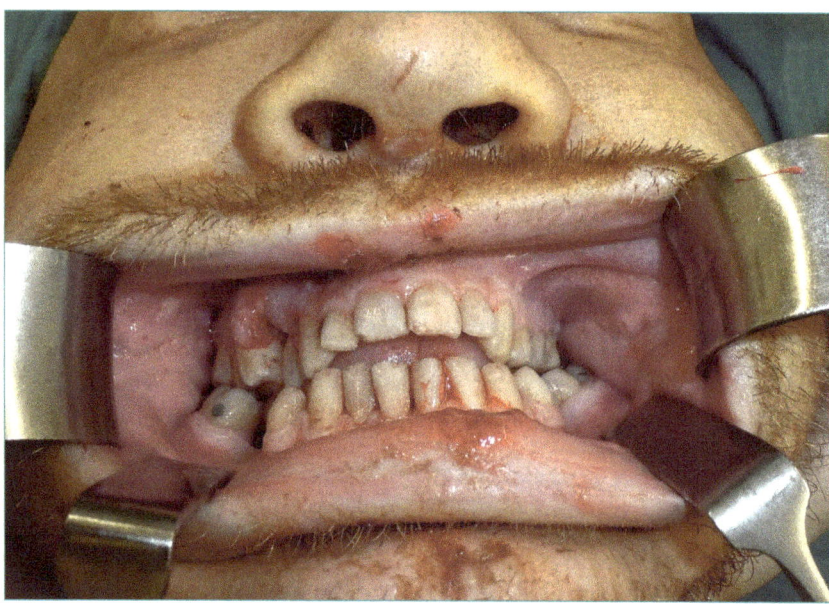

Figure 1.2: This gentleman presented with an altered occlusion. Notice how his front teeth are wide open, despite biting on his posterior teeth. This is called an 'anterior open bite' or 'AOB'. This is commonly seen in patients with Le Fort fractures. Picture courtesy of Mr. Madan Ethunandan

It is important to systematically assess the mucosal surfaces. These areas include:

- The buccal mucosa (inner lining of cheek), including the opening of the parotid duct opposite the upper second molar

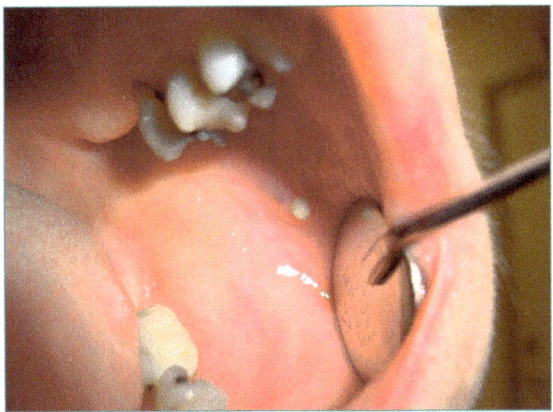

Figure 1.3: The parotid duct opens in the buccal mucosa opposite the upper second molar. Here it can be seen to discharging frank pus. This is usually indicative of parotitis. Picture courtesy of Mr. S Walsh

- The labial mucosa (inner surface of lips) and frenulum, which can be injured
- The lips themselves, including the presence of any numbness/altered sensation
- The gingival surfaces (gums) – including looking for gum boils (sinuses), as mentioned above

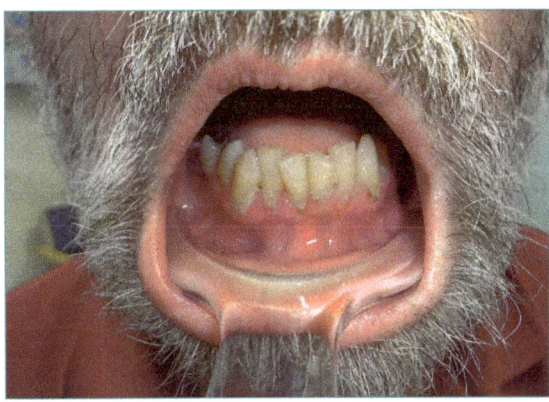

Figure 1.4: You can see that the gingivae of the lower front teeth looks acutely inflamed, with evidence of desquamation or 'sloughing'. This patient was being treated for pemphigus, a blistering condition. Picture courtesy of Mr. Stephen Walsh

- The hard palate
- The soft palate
- The tongue (dorsal surface, lateral border and ventral aspect)
- The floor of the mouth
- The oropharynx
- The retromolar region (area of mucosa just behind the last standing molar tooth).

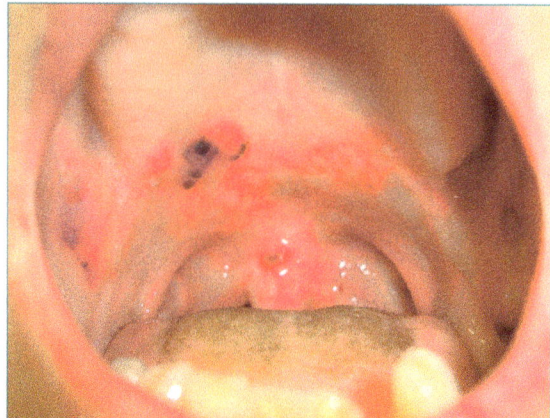

Figure 1.5: Here at the junction between the hard and the soft palate, the patient presented with acute blistering. Notice that on the right soft palate some of the blisters look like they are blood filled. This was mucous membrane pemphigoid. Picture courtesy of Mr. Stephen Walsh

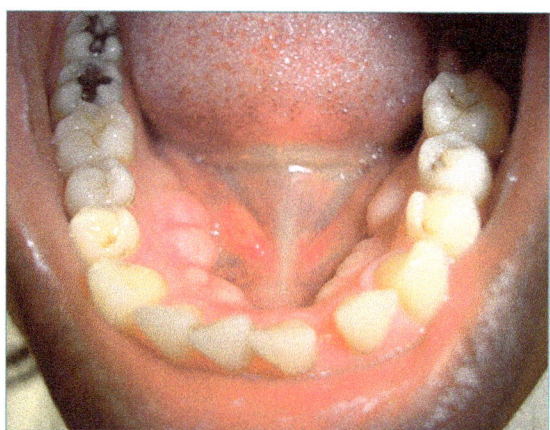

Figure 1.6: This patient presented with a mass in the right floor of the mouth. This was later found to be a salivary stone, which is just visible beneath the mucosal surface. The patient also presented with mandibular tori, bony exostoses that will be covered later in this book. Picture courtesy of Mr. Stephen Walsh

As with any lump or bump, any lesion (for example, a swelling or ulcer) found in the mouth should be assessed to establish its site, size, shape, colour and border, and for the presence of any associated (cervical) lymphadenopathy.

Neck Examination

The principles of a good neck examination will be familiar, and the standard inspection and palpation sequence should be followed. Observation might highlight any areas of concern, and examination of lumps and lesions can be described in terms of their site, size, shape, colour, consistency, nature of their borders and any trans-illumination (though this is rarely used in the head and neck). They are also assessed in relation to swallowing and tongue protrusion.

If a neck examination reveals lymphadenopathy, it is imperative to examine the skin, oral cavity, nose and face for potential sources of malignancy, and where appropriate, the other lymph-node sites (axilla, groin) and abdomen for signs of other lymphadenopathy or hepato-splenomegaly. We'll review this again in Chapter 5 where we look at neck lumps.

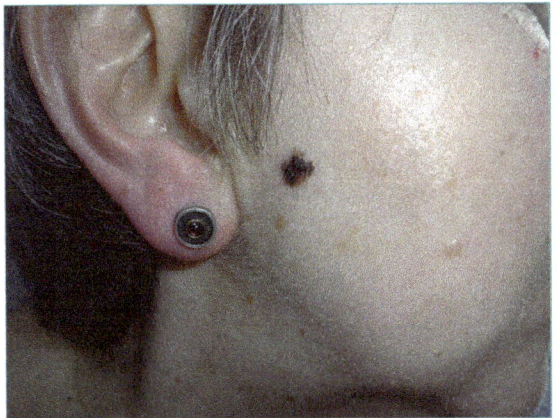

Figure 1.7: A patient presented with a change in a mole. Excisional biopsy identified this as malignant melanoma. Whilst less common than other forms of skin cancer, melanoma can present with lymphadenopathy in the head and neck. Picture courtesy of Mr. Stephen Walsh

Of course, depending on your findings, you might need to carry out more detailed examination of particular areas – for example, the eye, ear or cranial nerves. However, the examination framework above will hopefully be useful to help you better understand the information in the next chapters.

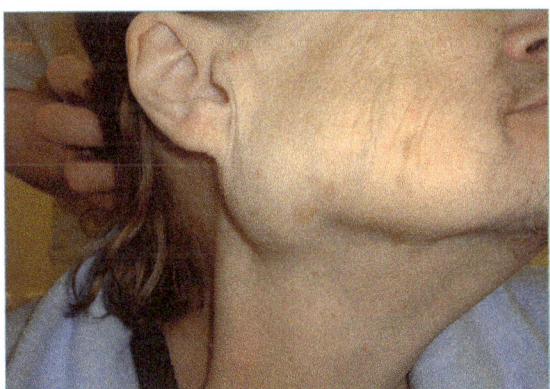

Figure 1.8: This patient was referred in with a right neck lump. A mass was identified in the right tail of the parotid. Most parotid masses are benign. Picture courtesy of Mr. Stephen Walsh

1.3 SOME IMPORTANT INVESTIGATIONS

Depending on your history and examination findings, further information is often gained through a variety of further investigations, ranging from simple blood tests to complex forms of imaging. Not all of these will be immediately available to you in a dental setting, and may require referral to the hospital directly or via the patient's GP.

8   ORAL AND MAXILLOFACIAL SURGERY

Head and neck imaging is complicated to interpret. As dental students, you will tend to be unfamiliar with soft-tissue imaging but will be well versed in the interpretation of the OPG and intra-oral periapical films. Increasingly, the use of cone beam CT scans (CBCT) is an area of learning for dental students and dental practitioners alike.

Plain Film Imaging

Below are examples of the three most common forms of plain radiograph image that help us better investigate and visualise the facial skeleton.

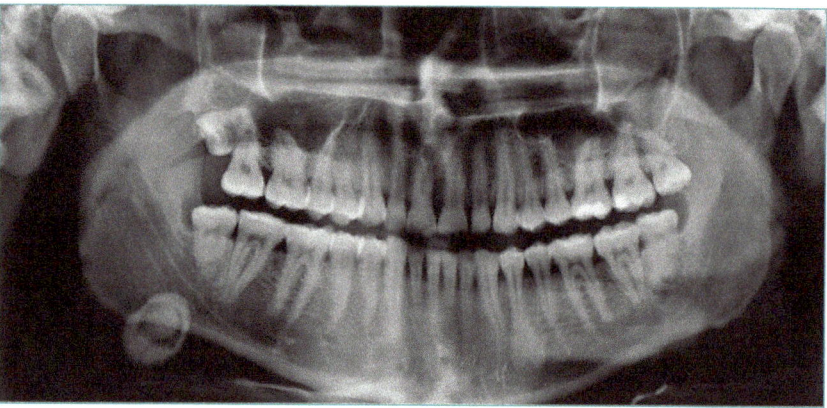

Figure 1.9: This is the most common radiograph used in OMFS. It is called an 'orthopantomogram'. It is a panoramic radiograph of the maxilla and mandible, showing all of the teeth, skeletal structures, maxillary sinuses and temporomandibular joints. It is useful for assessment of dental caries, abscesses, potential trauma or, as in this example, identifying submandibular stones. Picture courtesy of Mr. Stephen Walsh

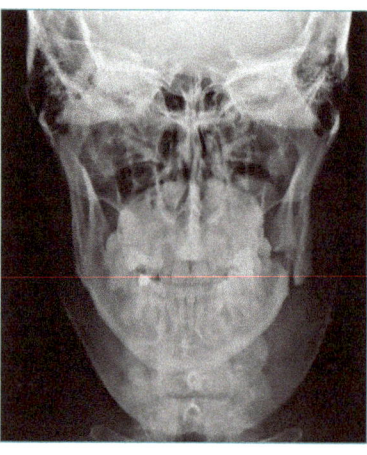

Figure 1.10: This is a 'PA mandible'. This, when combined with an OPG, can help identify fractures of the mandible. Here a fracture of the left angle of the mandible can be seen.

AN ILLUSTRATED GUIDE   9

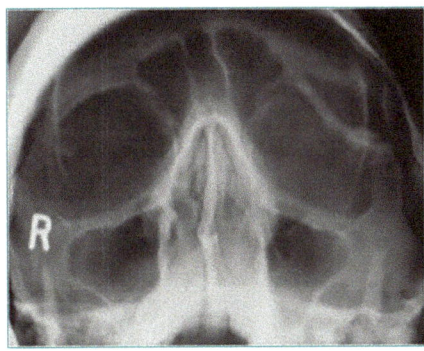

Figure 1.11: Occipitomental radiographs, commonly known as 'facial views', are useful for the assessment of the midface and peri-orbital regions in trauma patients. They can be challenging to interpret on first view, but the key is to draw a line down the middle of the face and to look for symmetry – or in this case, asymmetry! If you compare the right superior orbital rim with the left, you can see this patient has a left supra-orbital rim fracture involving the roof of the orbit. Picture courtesy of Mr. Graham Bounds

Over recent years, access to facial CT scans has improved. In particular, the ability rapidly to create, and then manipulate, 3D reformats and constructions for various facial structures have become extremely useful, in diagnosis, surgical planning and, of course, helping patients understand their own injuries.

In dental practice the most common use for CBCT scans is for the evaluation and assessment of patients requiring third-molar extractions or considerations for implants. It is beyond the remit of this textbook to help you learn how to evaluate CBCT scans, but these skills can be acquired after spending time within a maxillofacial unit either as a student or dental core trainee, or attending one of the many commercial courses available for interpretation.

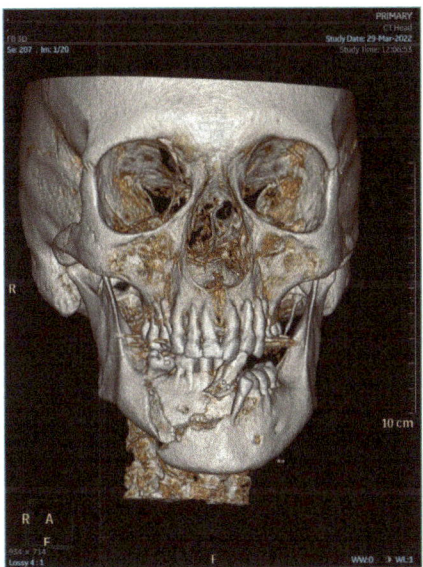

Figure 1.12: Extensively comminuted mandible sustained after a horse kick to the face. This 3D reformat is useful to visualise the injury and can be a useful aid for explaining to patients why teeth have to be lost. Picture courtesy of Miss Nabeela Ahmed

Blood Tests

When undertaking OMFS and Oral Medicine placements, some familiarity with the routine blood tests requested is advantageous, alongside an understanding of what is a normal result compared to an abnormal result.

We have listed the most commonly requested tests in our daily practice (with a brief explanation of why they are used), but obviously cannot cover the full spectrum of tests available. Each hospital will have a slightly different reference range for normal – hence values again haven't been listed.

Full Blood Count (FBC)

This covers haemoglobin, white-cell count, platelets and neutrophils, which are the most common reviewed parameters, but will also advise you the mean corpuscular haemoglobin (MCH) and mean corpuscular volume (MCV), which are useful when reviewing patients with low haemoglobin levels to ascertain whether this is an acute or chronic issue if the haemoglobin is low.

Urea and Electrolytes

This test evaluates how the kidneys are working. It includes urea and creatinine, and the electrolytes sodium and potassium. It can guide fluid resuscitation and prescription for those requiring intravenous fluid supplementation. This test is an important one to evaluate when prescribing medications that are renally excreted and may impair renal function when there is pre-existing renal disease.

Liver Function Tests

These give an overview of how the liver is functioning, and whether infection or medications are impinging on this function. They include albumin, ALP (alkaline phosphatase), ALT (alanine transaminase), AST (aspartate aminotransferase) and gamma-glutamyl transferase (GGT), which are all different enzymes made by the liver. It should also include bilirubin and lactate dehydrogenase (LD), other markers of liver function.

CRP

This is a test often requested when assessing patients for infection/inflammation in a more acute infection/sepsis setting. Alongside a raised WCC, this may guide you as to how unwell a patient presenting with infection may be.

ESR

Erythrocyte sedimentation rate – this is another test to evaluate the inflammatory process. Often used for assessment of systemic disease such as rheumatoid arthritis.

Clotting Screen

This test is an assessment of the intrinsic and extrinsic clotting pathways. Used for any patient presenting with a bleed, and who may be taking drugs that affect the clotting process such as warfarin.

Group and Save

This is a blood test taken for a patient who is bleeding (or may potentially bleed) and requires blood. This evaluates their blood group, so that if blood is required, the process to provide it will be faster.

Cross Match

This is a request for blood products, which will then be sourced from the regional blood blank – and mobilised to be available for the patient.

Haematinics – Vitamin B12, Folate, Ferritin and Zinc

These are often assessed together for patients presenting with oral ulceration, mucosal abnormality or a burning mouth/tongue. They can be deranged, and when identified, supplementation may impact significantly on symptoms.

This is just a small array of blood tests that you'll see being requested in OMFS outpatient clinics and ward rounds. Many hospitals will have electronic requesting processes, which simplifies the task of knowing which blood test tube is required for each test. This is something to observe when you attend the hospital for your maxillofacial placements.

1.4 THE TRAUMA PATIENT

While the incidence of both military and civilian wartime facial injuries has decreased, management of the trauma patient – usually due to interpersonal violence or road-traffic accidents – continues to represent a significant workload for oral and maxillofacial surgeons. It is useful to appreciate the role we play in the overall management of these patients.

As with all trauma patients, patients with facial trauma should be managed as per the Advanced Trauma Life Support (ATLS) algorithm (ABCDE: airway, breathing, circulation, disability, exposure), which is centred on quickly identifying and managing life-threatening injuries. Certain facial injuries are picked up during the primary survey and as such warrant immediate intervention. This usually takes place alongside the rest of the trauma team, in an effort to stem major bleeding (for example, in significant midface injuries) or maintain a threatened airway, using a surgical airway such as an immediate/emergency cricothyroidotomy (in a patient for whom emergency intubation fails and who cannot otherwise be ventilated) or elective tracheostomy (for a medium-term surgical airway).

Another important life-altering post-traumatic injury relates to bleeding around the eye. This is known as a retrobulbar haemorrhage, and unless treated urgently with a surgical decompression via a lateral canthotomy and cantholysis this can lead to blindness. Fortunately, this type of haemorrhage is rare, but it is an OMFS emergency.

Once these injuries have been addressed, patients are then assessed in a secondary survey, where it is more common to identify many of the typical facial injuries one would sustain in a traumatic event – fractures to the facial skeleton, lacerations, muscle and nerve injuries or dental trauma.

Assessing a trauma patient can be daunting and it is easy to get lost without a system to assess them. A commonly used measurement is the Glasgow Coma Score, which is scored out of 15 to evaluate patients with a head and facial injuries. The patient, if conscious, can be highly distressed, and their injuries can appear drastic. It is therefore even more important to be systematic. The framework laid out in this chapter will help you order your thoughts.

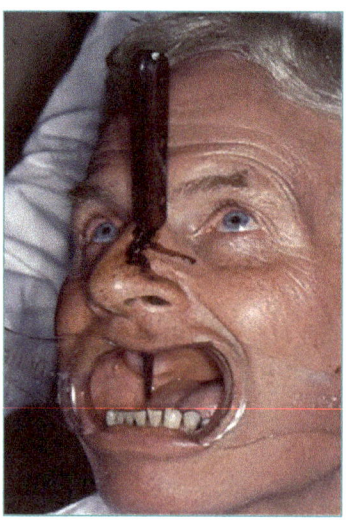

Figure 1.13: Approaching all trauma patients using ATLS principles is essential. Despite the dramatic presentation of this patient, considering the patient's airway, breathing and circulation is a cornerstone of managing this patient. Picture courtesy of Mr. Graham Bounds

CHAPTER 2: THE MOUTH

2.1 ANATOMY

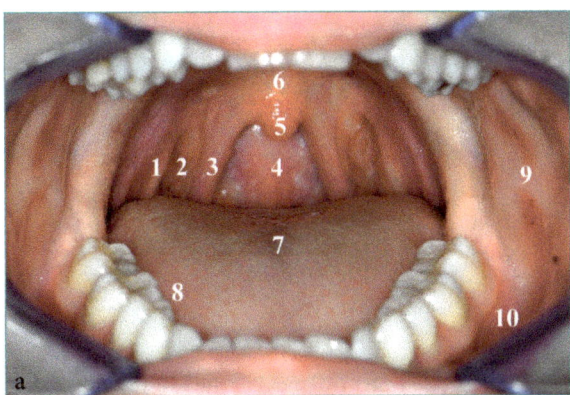

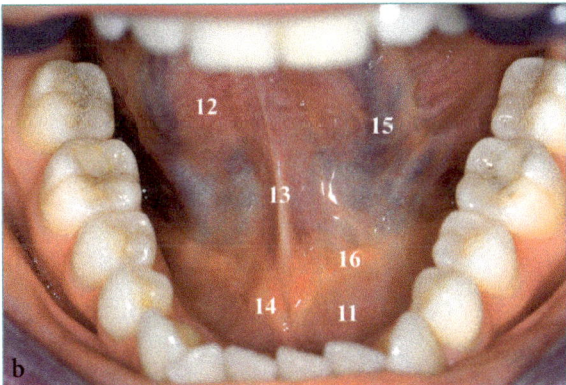

Figures 2.1a & Figures 2.1b: Intraoral and b) floor of mouth anatomy. The parotid duct drains via the parotid papilla, which is out of sight, opposite the upper second molar teeth bilaterally:

1. *Palatoglossal arch*
2. *Palatine tonsil*
3. *Palatopharyngeal arch*
4. *Posterior pharyngeal wall*
5. *Uvula*
6. *Soft palate*
7. *Dorsum of tongue*
8. *Lateral border of tongue*
9. *Buccal mucosa*
10. *Buccal sulcus*
11. *Floor of mouth*
12. *Ventral surface of tongue*
13. *Lingual fraenum*
14. *Submandibular duct openings*
15. *Lingual vein*
16. *Sublingual fold*

2.2 ULCERS AND PATCHES IN THE MOUTH

Wherever it is on the body, an ulcer is simply a break in the continuity of the epithelial surface due to progressive tissue destruction. In the mouth, it is important clinically to examine an ulcer's appearance and site, and note the history of its occurrence. Self-limiting, recurrent or relapsing–remitting ulcers are often caused by different (typically inflammatory) aetiologies than persistent ulcers (those which appear and never go away), which are far more likely to be malignant.

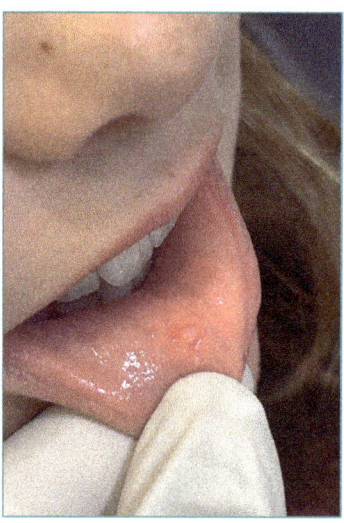

Figure 2.2: Benign aphthous ulcer. Typical small, shallow-looking ulcer with a well-defined margin seen here on the ventral aspect of the left tongue. Picture courtesy of Miss Nabeela Ahmed

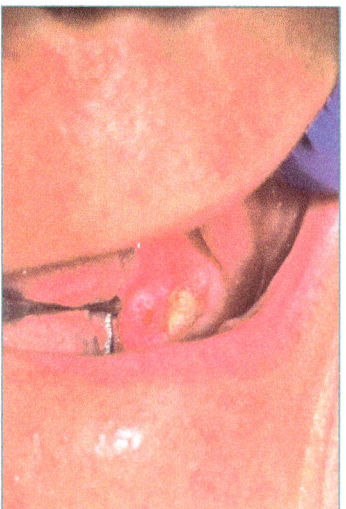

Figure 2.3: This is a malignant lesion. It has a speckled look and an irregular margin, and is raised towards the lingual aspect where it is ulcerated. Picture courtesy of Miss Nabeela Ahmed

FACT BOX

When investigating the cause of an ulcer, one must consider the following factors:
- Risk-factor assessment:
  - Smoker?
  - Alcohol intake?
- Painful vs. painless
- Duration (< or >3 weeks?)
- Persistent vs. recurrent
- Solitary or multiple
- Previous history of oral cancer
- Medication associated?
  - Nicorandil
  - Aspirin
- Associations with other systemic symptoms:
  - Ulcers in other areas (e.g. skin, genital, corneal)
  - History of autoimmune disease

SINISTER FEATURES:
- Extending beyond mucosa
- Irregular border
- Firm/indurated
- Associated neck lymphadenopathy – single or more than one node
- Nerve weakness/altered sensation
- Not healed after three weeks
- On high-risk areas (lateral tongue, floor of mouth, retromolar, etc.)
- Painless ulcer
- Loose/missing/deviated teeth
- Previous oral-cancer history
- Risk-factor history (smoking, excessive alcohol consumption, betel-nut chewing)

2.2.1 SUSPICIOUS ULCERS

Oral cancers, most usually squamous cell carcinomas (SCC), often present as a persistent, yet relatively painless, firm and indurated ulcer (present for more than three weeks). These ulcers aren't like a normal aphthous ulcer, which are small (around 2–3mm) and painful; they are destructive and will spread beyond the soft mucosal surfaces onto the firmer gingiva and into deeper tissues (sometimes you will see necrotic muscle/fat/bone at the base). As the cancer invades surrounding nerve fibres, a once-painful ulcer may become surprisingly painless. If a cancer invades a named peripheral nerve (such as the inferior alveolar nerve or hypoglossal nerve), symptoms like lower-lip numbness or asymmetrical tongue protrusion might be found on examination. Bone tends to be invaded later and may lead to loose teeth or even fracture of the jaw – beware of a patient with unexplainably loose teeth next to a swelling or persistent mouth ulcer! Irregular shape and, most importantly, induration (palpable firmness) should raise suspicion for cancer, as should the presence of firm, palpable lymph nodes in the neck.

2.2.2 BENIGN ORAL ULCERATION

Benign persistent ulceration may be secondary to a persistent insult or irritation to the mucosa. This is commonly seen with chronic local trauma: for example, mucosa rubbing against a sharp tooth or dental filling can, over time, lead to erosion and ulceration of the tissue. It will persist or worsen until the cause is removed (via smoothing of the sharp surface). Some topical irritants

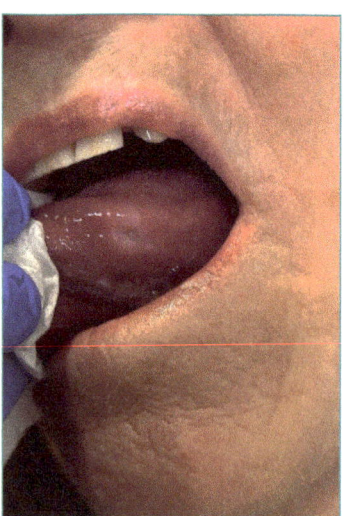

Figure 2.4: This is a traumatic ulcer caused by a sharp tooth. Once the sharp tooth is addressed, the ulcer will disappear. Picture courtesy of Mr. Madan Ethunandan

such as aspirin used directly onto mouth tissue can cause a chemical burn which destroys the tissue. In some cases, oral ulceration can be a recognised side effect of systemic medications, such as nicorandil.

2.2.3 RECURRENT ULCERATION

In the absence of systemic disease, recurrent ulceration – often termed 'recurrent aphthous stomatitis' (RAS) – is one of the commonest presentations and has affected up to 50% of the population at some stage or another. These ulcers can present during times of stress, including exams. RAS generally presents in three clinical forms: major RAS, minor RAS and herpetiform.

Benign recurrent oral ulceration can also be secondary to systemic autoimmune disease such as pemphigus, pemphigoid and Bechet's disease. You may come across these in dermatology or autoimmune clinics.

Patients with suspected RAS should be investigated for nutritional deficiency (haematinics including iron studies, vitamin B12 and folate, as well as zinc levels should be evaluated). Psychological stress, as with gastric ulcers, can cause mouth ulcers, so these potential causes should be looked into in the first instance. Once these simpler causes are ruled out, a trial of Difflam™ (benzydamine) mouthwash (which has a mild local-anaesthetic action) with or without a steroid mouthwash (e.g. prednisolone or betamethasone) can be initiated. Topical hydrocortisone steroid pellets placed on the ulcer can be very effective as well.

2.2.4 ERYTHEMA MULTIFORME

This is an immune mediated condition of rapid onset that may present to the dental surgeon. It can be triggered by viral infection or medication or may arise spontaneously with no obvious cause. When triggered by an obvious precipitant it is referred to as Stevens Johnson Syndrome. As you can appreciate from Figure 2.5, it can be incredibly painful and described as blistering and peeling of the oral mucosal membranes. Depending on its severity it may merit admission to hospital and management with removal/avoidance of the causative trigger and supportive measures (as patients may be unable to eat and drink) using intravenous fluids, antibiotics and steroids whilst the mucosal membranes recover. You may wish to liaise with the local dermatology service for support as there may be widespread skin and other mucosal membrane involvement, and if not treated rapidly can become life threatening. When you see a patient with rapid onset of oral mucosal ulceration, please consider this diagnosis.

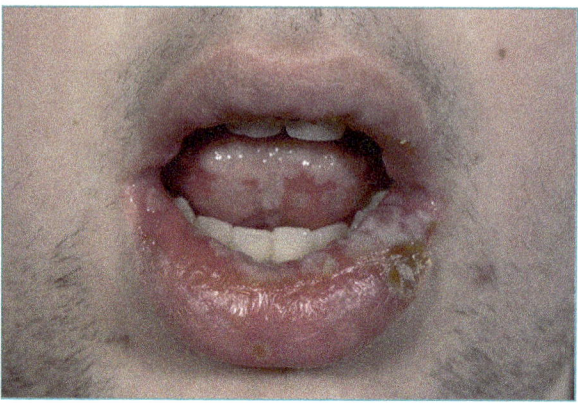

Figure 2.5: Picture of extensive oral ulceration of rapid onset affecting the lips and tongue in a patient with erythema multiforme. Picture courtesy of Mr. Andrew Sidebottom

2.2.5 PATCHES

Patches in the mouth are usually white, brown-pigmented, red or a mixture. Some types are more likely to be premalignant (known as severe dysplasia or carcinoma-in-situ) or frankly malignant (invasive cancer). They are often flat/macular in nature. Clinical diagnosis can be challenging, based on visual appearance alone. Here, we divide patches into 'mainly red', 'mainly white' and 'pigmented'.

In general, redness indicates a degree of epithelial atrophy or thinning of the mucosa (which may eventually lead to erosion/ulceration). A red patch of unknown origin (erythroplakia) is suspicious for premalignancy/malignant change and warrants urgent investigation.

A white patch that does not rub off gently with a tongue depressor often indicates a 'thickening' of the epithelium, due to increased production of keratin. This keratosis may occur as a protective response against repeated trauma, to strengthen the mucosa; however, it may represent premalignant change. There should be a low threshold for subsequent investigation. Where there is no identifiable cause, a tenacious white patch in the mouth is called 'leukoplakia' and may well be a premalignant lesion. *Leukoplakia is a white patch which cannot be diagnosed as anything else following investigation.*

Oral submucous fibrosis (OSMF) is a premalignant condition associated with betel-nut chewing. Betel nut is combined with other agents including tobacco and slaked lime to form gutkha (or paan). This is a habit common, but not exclusive, to South Asian cultures. It presents with a pale, scarred appearance to the buccal (cheek) mucosa, making it rigid and restricting mouth opening.

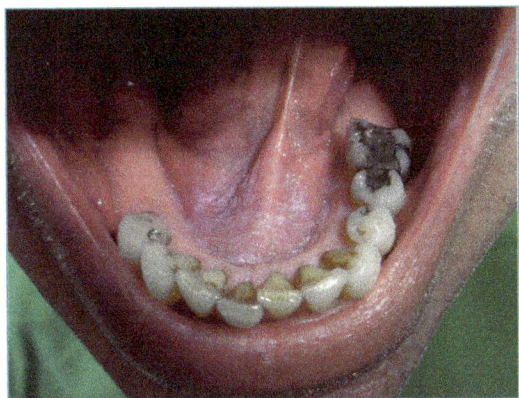

Figure 2.6: This patient presented with a white patch in the floor of the mouth. Incisional biopsy confirmed this was a keratosis. Picture courtesy of Mr. Stephen Walsh

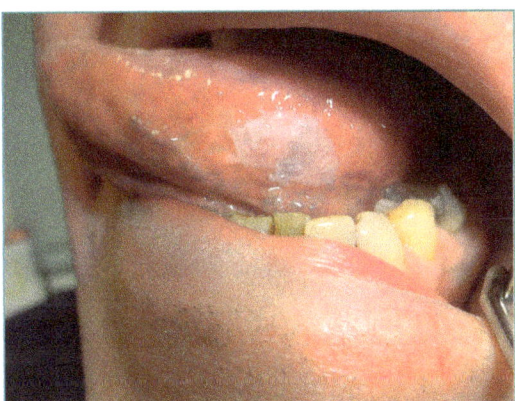

Figure 2.7: This patient presented with a white patch on the left lateral tongue. This would not rub away and there was no identifiable cause. This is therefore called a 'leukoplakia'. A biopsy is the next step in establishing a diagnosis. Picture courtesy of Mr. Stephen Walsh

White Patches

Oral lichen planus (LP) typically (but not exclusively) presents with symmetrically bilateral lesions on the mucosa/tongue/gingiva. Its appearance can be variable and up to six types have been classified.

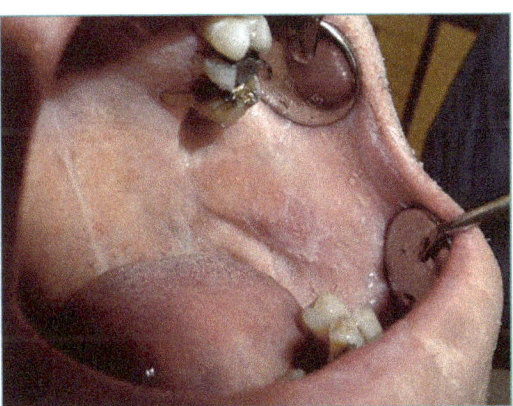

Figure 2.8: This patient presented with lichen planus in the left buccal mucosa. Picture courtesy of Mr. Madan Ethunandan

Patients may present with no symptoms, or experience soreness and discomfort in the area when eating/drinking certain foods (e.g. spicy food). Furthermore, this condition can present with involvement of other epithelial sites (eyes, skin, genital mucosa), which may point to a systemic condition requiring input from other specialities (e.g. gynaecology for vulvovaginal LP). Lichen planus is a T-lymphocyte-mediated disorder and is thought to have malignant potential, so getting the diagnosis by incisional biopsy is important as it may have life-long implications. Treatment varies according to disease severity, from a simple steroid mouthwash and other topical applications, to systemic immunosuppressive medications.

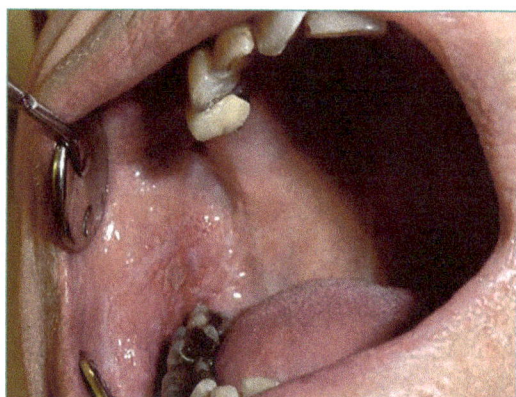

Figure 2.9: *This is a form of lichen planus known as erosive LP. Patients may be asymptomatic or may be in varying levels of pain. Picture courtesy of Mr. Madan Ethunandan*

Lichenoid reactions have a similar clinical and identical histopathological appearance to LP (although it is commonly asymmetrically distributed in the mouth) and is secondary to outside causes (drugs, heavy-metal fillings or even a change in toothpaste). The aim of management is to identify and remove the offending cause, as well as relieving symptoms in a similar fashion to LP.

Candida infection can result in a localised white pseudomembranous coating of the epithelial surface. A white patch that easily wipes off with a tongue depressor is highly suggestive of pseudomembranous candidiasis and should respond promptly and completely to antifungal treatments such as fluconazole or topical nystatin. It is often worth asking a patient if they wear their dentures all the time, or if they are using a steroid inhaler, which are common causes of acute infection. Chronic candida infection as seen in chronic hyperplastic candidiasis (thickened candida-infected mucosa with a white appearance that doesn't scrape off) does, however, have malignant potential. Patients with this condition need to be monitored and are often treated with regular courses of potent oral antifungal tablets such as fluconazole.

One of the most common benign causes of a white patch in the mouth is frictional keratosis, where chronic mechanical trauma (e.g. cheek biting) can lead to a thickening (and therefore whitening) of the epithelium, as a protective measure. This is similar to hard skin on the soles of the feet through heavy walking. If you put your feet into water, this hard skin turns white due to waterlogging. Hard skin in the mouth is constantly bathed by saliva! This diagnosis should only be made if there is an obvious cause – for example, a rough dental filling, a sharp tooth rubbing on the affected area or a white thickening of the buccal mucosa in-line with the occlusal plane can cause this frictional keratosis.

Some white patches can be a completely physiological phenomenon, such as Fordyce spots and leukoedema – a bluish/white hue of the mucosa, more commonly found in people with darker skin pigmentation. But this is fine-print stuff for the non-specialist.

Red Patches

Geographic tongue (also known as benign migratory glossitis) has a characteristic 'world-map-like' morphology, occurring on the dorsum of the tongue. Its cause is unknown. Although it results in alternating areas of sore, red, atrophic mucosa with characteristic pale halo-like borders, it is entirely benign and there is no known link with premalignancy or cancer. Diagnosis is made on clinical examination only.

Another benign red patch is the red atrophic changes commonly related to an underlying infection such as oral candidiasis, particularly seen in denture

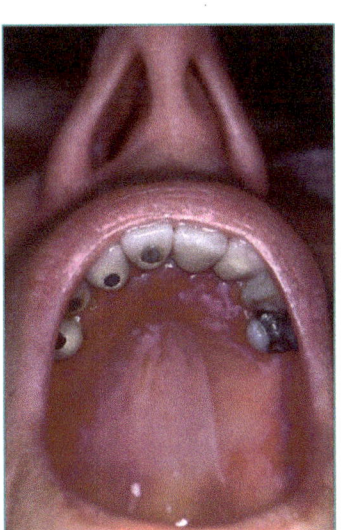

Figure 2.10: This is a typical presentation oral candidiasis due to inadequate denture hygiene. You can see the erythema fits beautifully within the limits where the partial denture normally sits. You can actually see the outline perfectly! Picture courtesy of Mr. Andrew Sidebottom

wearers. This is the result of inadequate hygiene – simple denture care and topical and/or oral antifungals can resolve the situation within days. The clinical picture is of a red patch confined to the mucosa that is in direct contact with the underside of the denture – essentially a size-matched 'print' of the denture fitting surface.

Angular cheilitis is a bacterial or fungal infection which can present as a sore red or cracked area that does not heal, most commonly in the corner of the lips. Similarly, candida infection of the tongue can present with a classical midline red patch on the dorsum of the tongue, known as median rhomboid glossitis (MRG) due to its diamond shape. This is treated with a short course of topical and/or systemic antifungal treatment such as fluconazole. However, should atrophic candida infections fail to resolve with appropriate treatment, erythroplakia (and therefore premalignancy) remains a high possibility, warranting urgent investigation.

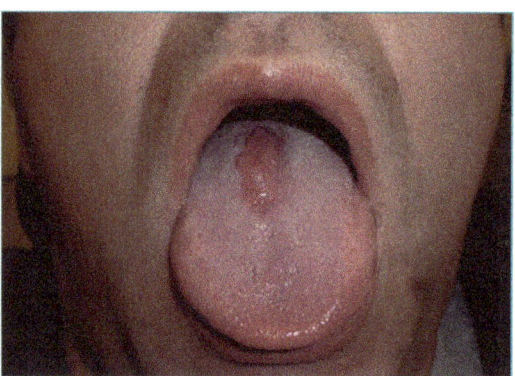

Figure 2.11: This is a classic presentation of median rhomboid glossitis. It responds well to antifungal medications. Picture courtesy of Miss Nabeela Ahmed

Pigmented Lesions

Pigmented (blue/brown) lesions in the mouth are common and often arise through 'tattooing' of the mucosa from an existing or previous amalgam dental filling. Despite this, mucosal melanoma (although very rare) is a diagnosis not to be missed. A common cause of a brown midline patch of the tongue is 'black hairy tongue'. In itself, this is a benign condition where overgrowth of the filiform papillae (taste buds) traps pigment from food, bacteria and yeast, leading to discolouration. It can be improved by using a toothbrush to scrub the area with a bicarbonate-based toothpaste. A similarly named condition that is different in appearance is called 'oral hairy leukoplakia' of the tongue. This is caused by Epstein-Barr virus (EBV), and may be a presenting feature of HIV infection or immunosuppression. It is characterised by fine, white, corrugated ('hairy') lines typically on the lateral edges of the tongue.

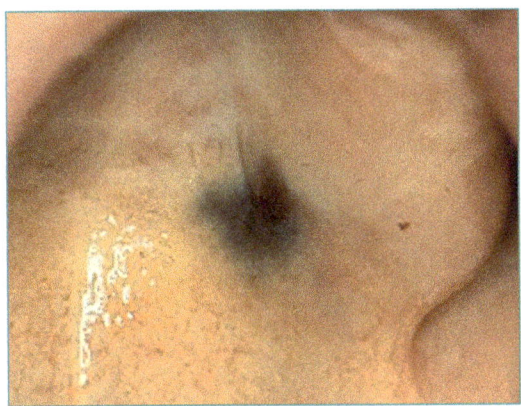

Figure 2.12: Amalgam tattoo on the palatal mucosa. These are most commonly seen in the buccal/labial sulcus and can be confirmed by taking a periapical x-ray, where the amalgam fleck/s can often be seen. Picture courtesy of Professor Peter Brennan

Pigmented lesions tend to be blue or black in colour. Importantly, whilst incredibly rare, representing less than 1% of head and neck melanoma, mucosal melanoma must be a consideration and should be considered in the differential diagnosis. Some systemic disorders, for example Addison's disease or Peutz-Jeghers syndrome (see Figure 2.13), can present with brown pigmented patches in the oral cavity.

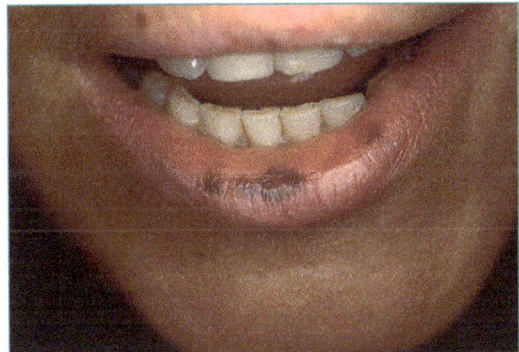

Figure 2.13: Picture of Peutz-Jeghers pigmentation of lower lip. There can be a manifestation of this condition which pre-disposes to hamartomatous polyps of the bowel. Picture courtesy of Mr. Andrew Sidebottom

2.3 LUMPS AND SWELLINGS IN THE MOUTH

> **SINISTER FEATURES:**
> - A lump in the upper lip and soft palate is malignant until proven otherwise
> - Associated ulceration
> - Fixity to deep tissues
> - Irregular border
> - Lymphadenopathy
> - Nerve weakness/altered sensation of the tongue or lip/cheek
> - On high-risk areas (lateral tongue, floor of mouth, retromolar)
> - Previous oral cancer
> - Rapidly growing
> - Strong risk-factor history (smoking, alcohol, betel-nut chewing)

Malignant Causes of Swelling

In all presentations of a 'lump in the mouth', cancer must be ruled out first and foremost. Oral cancer is discussed in section 2.4 in more detail. Squamous cell carcinoma (SCC) is the commonest type of mouth cancer and typically presents as a non-healing ulcer which then becomes indurated and fixed to underlying structures, eventually taking on the form of a 'lump'. Salivary-gland tumours may also occur in the mouth. The site of a salivary-gland tumour has a significant influence on the likelihood of it being malignant – a general point to remember is that **the smaller the gland, the greater the chance of malignancy**. Lumps in the upper lip and the junction of the hard and soft palate are particularly risky; they are therefore presumed malignant until proven otherwise.

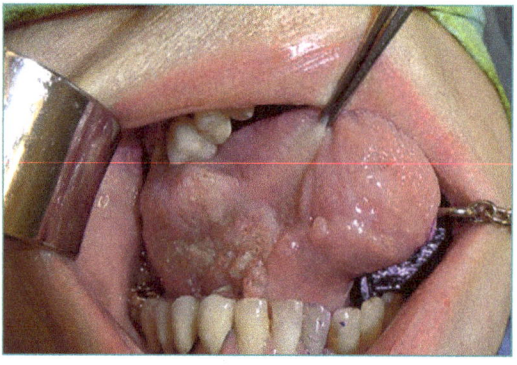

Figure 2.14: This patient presented with an advanced oral cancer. This would require an extensive resection, neck dissection and reconstruction, often with free-tissue transfer otherwise known as 'free flaps'. Picture courtesy of Mr. Madan Ethunandan

Malignant jaw tumours may be primary or secondary/metastatic in origin. Whilst SCCs arising in the mouth and invading into bone are the most common, metastasis of distant tumours to the craniofacial skeleton also occurs, as with metastases to other bones in the body (from the breast, lung, kidney, thyroid, colon or prostate). Rarely, malignant primary bone tumours may be odontogenic in origin (from tooth tissue), such as ameloblastic carcinoma, though as mentioned these are very rare in comparison to SCC.

Benign Causes of Swelling

Infection

Dental abscesses are one of the most common causes of benign/acute swelling in the mouth. Infection of a tooth leads to the accumulation of pus at the root tip, which in turn can track along the path of least resistance to the gingival surface. This presents as a dental sinus or 'gum boil'. The patient will commonly present with dental pain and teeth with associated periapical infection will be tender to percussion (tapping with the end of a metal instrument). This requires definitive treatment by a dentist, in the form of root canal treatment or extraction.

Fibroepithelial polyp

In the absence of an obvious dental infection, a fleshy mobile lump on the gingiva or mucosa is commonly a fibroepithelial polyp. These are believed to be caused by a form of chronic irritation, be that occlusal trauma to the cheek or persistent rubbing of a denture.

Diagnosis can usually be achieved by examination alone; however, histological assessment can provide definitive confirmation. As such, these lesions are treated by excisional biopsy and are often done for patient comfort.

Something very similar is seen in patients with dentures, where chronic irritation due to the rubbing of the edge of an ill-fitting denture can cause the formation of a painless, often lobulated mass. This is instead called 'denture-induced hyperplasia'. It is treated the same way as a fibroepithelial polyp, with the addition of adjusting the denture to prevent the ongoing source of irritation.

Mucocele/ranula

A mucocele is a collection of saliva in the oral mucosa caused by damage to a minor salivary gland. It commonly presents as a small localised translucent swelling in the lower lip which will repeatedly rupture and recur. A ranula is a generally larger mucocele of the floor of the mouth and, by definition, arises due to damage to the sublingual gland. Mucoceles are generally harmless

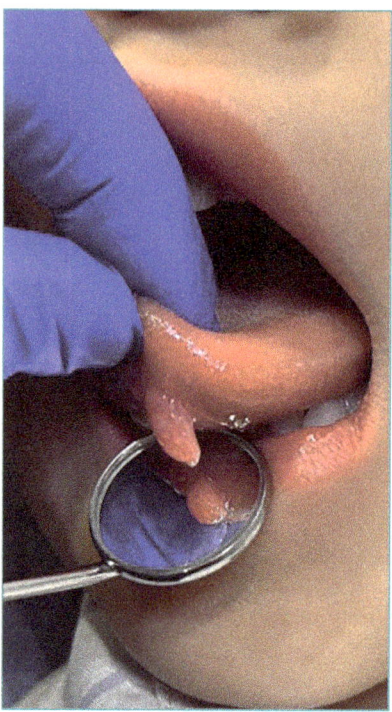

Figure 2.15: Picture of a fibroepithelial polyp/leaf fibroma. Picture courtesy of Miss Nabeela Ahmed

but can become infected and can also be a nuisance to patients, especially as they expand to become very large. These can therefore usually be managed by simple excision under local anaesthetic or, for the more stubborn lesions, excision of the affected sublingual gland. Remember – upper-lip lumps are more likely to be neoplastic or cancerous and always warrant investigation.

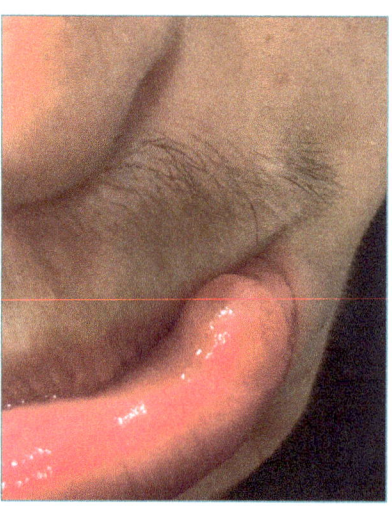

Figure 2.16: Picture of a mucocele of the left lower lip. Photo courtesy of Miss Nabeela Ahmed

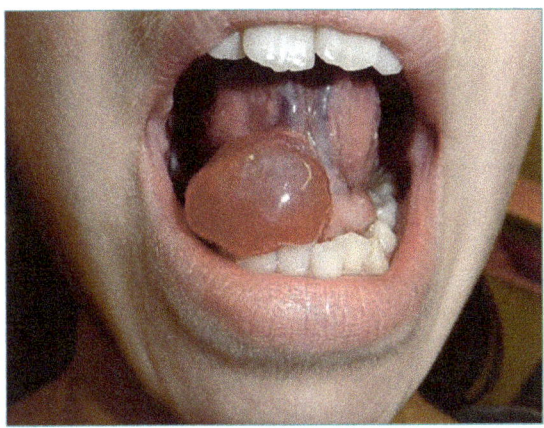

Figure 2.17: This is a ranula, a collection of saliva in the floor of the mouth. Sometimes they can herniate into the neck, otherwise known as a plunging ranula. Picture courtesy of Mr. Madan Ethunandan

Bony exostosis — tori

A simple hard lump of the mandible or maxilla is often described as a 'torus'. These are physiological bony outgrowths (exostoses) of indefinite duration (for as long as the patient can remember) usually found as either a symmetrical smooth midline swelling of the hard palate or bilateral symmetrical smooth swellings of the mandible, most often inside the jaw (on the lingual side), but can occur in either jaw.

Without any sinister features or ambiguity over the clinical diagnosis, these lesions can be monitored. Any change in its appearance, however, would suggest a pathological swelling and warrants further assessment. They may warrant surgical intervention if they compromise the use of a denture.

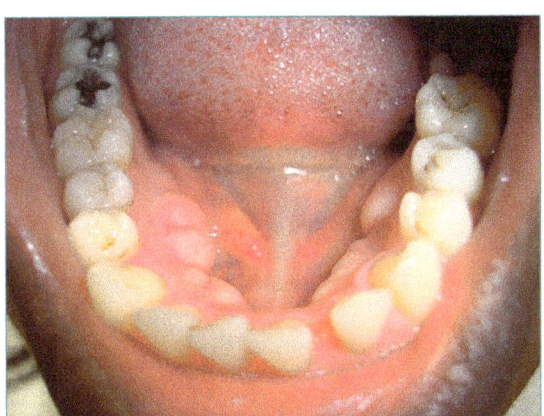

Figure 2.18: This is a classic picture of bilateral lingual tori. They appear as smooth, hard swellings. Picture courtesy of Mr. Stephen Walsh

2.4 ORAL CANCER

In the last thirty years there have been incredible advances in patient education, diagnosis and subsequent management of oral and oropharyngeal cancer, yet this has only been met with a minor improvement in the survival of patients. This remains attributed to late presentation.

Squamous Cell Carcinoma (SCC)

As with any cancer, the development of SCC is a multi-step process involving a cascade of oncogenes and the failure of tumour suppressor genes, of which p53 is the most commonly acknowledged.

The most well-known causes are tobacco smoking and alcohol, which have a synergistic effect (in other words, the harmful effect of these two risk factors combined is more harmful than simply the sum of their individual effects). The long-term use of betel nut (gutkha) can also lead to SCC in oral submucous fibrosis. Other, rarer causes include: a diet low in antioxidants and vitamins A and C; trauma; and infection (EBV and syphilis).

Human papilloma viruses (HPV) 16 and 18 spread by the genito-oral route have also become directly implicated in the development of not only oropharyngeal (tonsil and base-of-tongue cancers) but also (less commonly) SCCs limited to the oral cavity alone. Consequently, the disease is now presenting in younger adults and with greater balance between genders. The HPV vaccination now offered to both male and female school-age children is thought to have a protective effect against developing HPV-related head and neck cancers.

Assessment and Staging

The presentation of mouth cancers is described in section 2.3. Once a suspicious lesion is identified, confirmation of the diagnosis is by an incisional biopsy (typically under local anaesthetic), which also gives some idea about the tumour aggressiveness, followed by tumour staging. The latter involves clinical examination and cross-sectional imaging to give more detail regarding the presence of local, regional and distant spread of disease. Imaging typically includes one or more of the following:

- CT neck and thorax with IV contrast (scanning from the skull base down to the diaphragm; this highlights the primary tumour in the mouth, any involved lymph nodes in the neck and any likely lung metastases)
- Ultrasound-guided core biopsy (or fine-needle aspiration) of any palpable neck lumps

- MRI to evaluate for spread along nerves and involvement of bone marrow of the jaws.

For some small tumours with no evidence of regional or distant spread, and in cases where we don't need access to the neck to allow for reconstruction with free-tissue transfer, sentinel lymph node biopsy (SLNB) should be offered to the patient. This involves the use of radiotracer dyes that are injected into the primary tumour, combined with the use of an intra-operative gamma camera (radiation sensor) to locate and biopsy the first-draining ('first echelon' or 'sentinel') lymph node. This method helps to determine whether or not neck dissection surgery is needed, or just a simple excision of the mouth tumour. Some surgeons use this staging technique routinely, while others do not, for fear of missing spread of cancer to other lymph nodes in the neck (which is reported to occur in about 20–30% of small oral SCCs). For this reason, some surgeons even suggest that all (even the smallest) oral SCCs should be treated with elective neck dissection as this is proven to increase disease-specific survival (avoiding death from the mouth cancer) and overall survival (avoiding death for any reason). There are ongoing trials to evaluate this, so it is worthwhile asking what the approach is in your local maxillofacial unit.

Like other cancers in the body, oral/mouth cancers are staged with the TNM system:

T – describes the primary **t**umour,
N – describes the regional-lymph-**n**ode involvement, and
M – describes the presence or absence of distant **m**etastases.

This gives the multidisciplinary team (MDT) an idea of the extent of the disease, treatment needs and prognosis.

Treatment

In the mouth, surgery is the mainstay of cancer treatment. Primary radiotherapy (using radiotherapy as the main treatment) can be considered in some instances, but generally, it is used less commonly than other modalities due to its associated morbidity and the associated difficulty with patient compliance over a typical six-week course. Even with surgical treatment, postoperative radiotherapy may still be required for large and/or aggressive cancers.

Because of the variety of ways in which oral cancers can present anatomically and because most oral cancers present in a later stage (T3 or T4), cancer surgery performed by oral and maxillofacial surgeons is typically variable. This commonly requires aggressive major surgery to remove all tumour tissue with a surrounding safety margin of normal tissue (to ensure nothing is left behind in the adjacent structures), in combination with neck dissection to remove any further disease which has spread to the lymph nodes in the neck.

The extensiveness of such surgery means that a temporary tracheostomy tube (surgically inserted into the airway/trachea) is often performed at the beginning of the surgery to protect the patient's airway from bleeding and swelling in the immediate postoperative period. Furthermore, because of the large volume of tissue removed (and the impact upon facial aesthetics and oral functions such as chewing and swallowing), complex reconstructions are often needed. In current practice, this usually means that a pair of oral and maxillofacial surgeons perform the surgery together. One will remove the cancer while, at the same time, the second surgeon harvests tissue from elsewhere on the body to auto-transplant it into the head and neck region. This involves re-vascularising it by anastomosing (sewing together) the small 2–3mm diameter artery and vein(s) of the transplanted tissue to arteries and veins in the neck, under a surgical microscope. This is known as free-tissue (or free-flap) reconstruction and is performed in almost all UK head and neck cancer centres.

Oral and maxillofacial surgeons who perform major free-flap reconstructions regularly use a variety of flaps, depending upon the type of tissue that needs to be replaced. This may simply involve the replacement of soft tissue only (for example, using a radial forearm free flap or anterolateral thigh flap) or in more complex reconstructions, the replacement of both soft tissue and bone (for example, using free flaps of the fibula, scapula or iliac crest to reconstruct large defects of the facial skeleton or skull base).

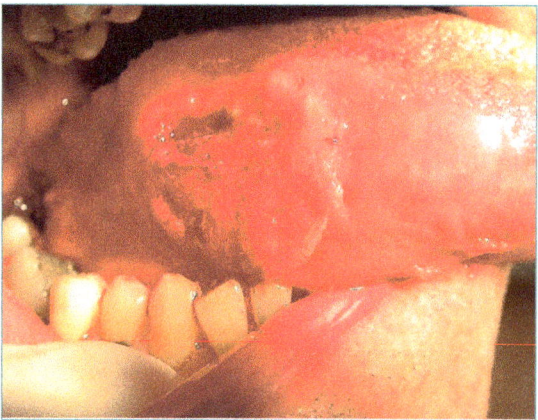

Figure 2.19: This patient presented with a biopsy-confirmed SCC of the right lateral tongue. As well as requiring a neck dissection, treatment would have consisted of resection of a large portion of the right side of the tongue. Picture courtesy of Professor P. Brennan

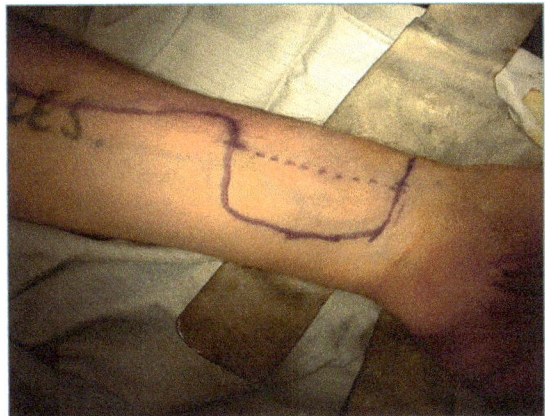

Figure 2.20: In order to restore form and function, and to aid speech, eating and swallowing, a radial forearm free flap from the patient's non-dominant arm would have been raised. Here you can see the surgeon's markings prior to commencing surgery. Picture courtesy of Professor P. Brennan

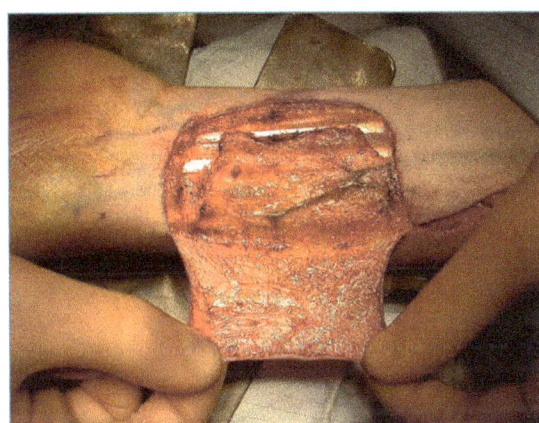

Figure 2.21: Here you can see the surgeon raising the flap. Notice the tendons of palmaris longus and flexor carpi radialis! Pictures courtesy of Professor P. Brennan

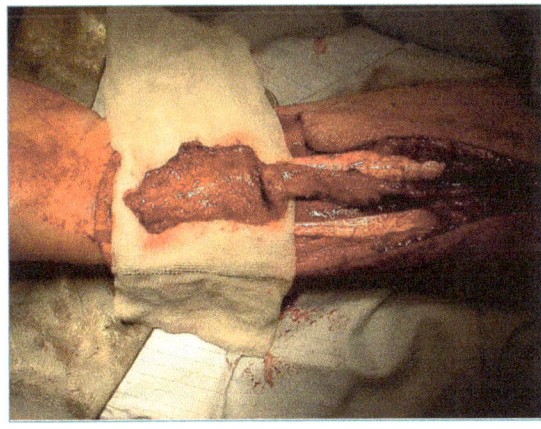

Figure 2.22: Here, the flap is fully raised. You can see the blood supply or 'pedicle' attached and travelling up to the patient's elbow, where it would later be disconnected prior to transfer to the neck for anastomosis. Picture courtesy of Professor P. Brennan

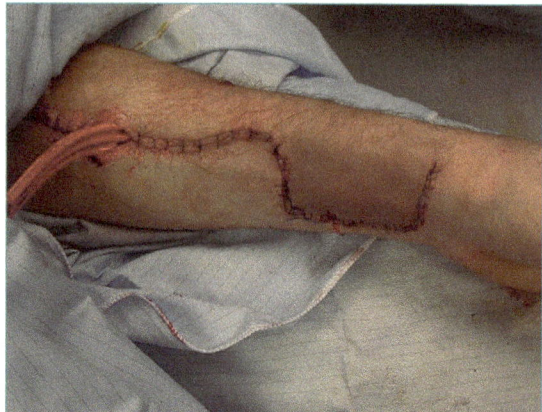

The donor site is closed. All surgeons will use drains and monitor the limb for any signs of vascular or neurological compromise. Picture courtesy of Professor P. Brennan

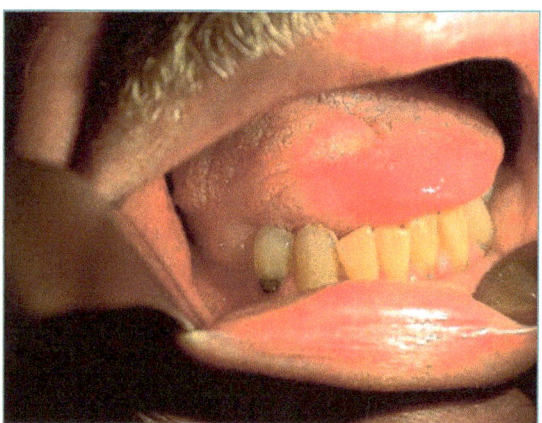

Figure 2.24: This is the patient six months post-surgery. Look how well the radial forearm free flap has integrated. It actually looks like a tongue! Picture courtesy of Professor P. Brennan

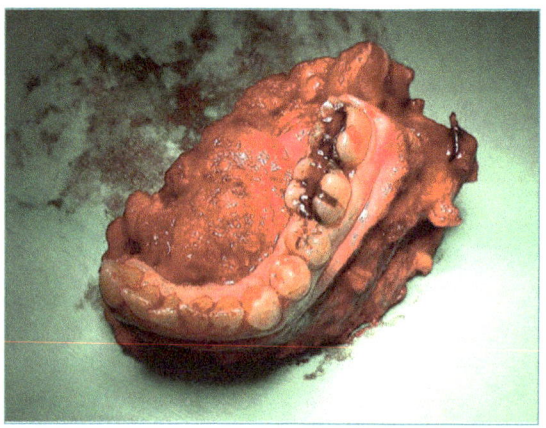

Figure 2.25: This patient presented with an extensive floor-of-mouth SCC invading the mandible. In order to achieve surgical clearance of the tumour, part of the patient's mandible needed to be resected as part of the specimen. Picture courtesy of Professor P. Brennan

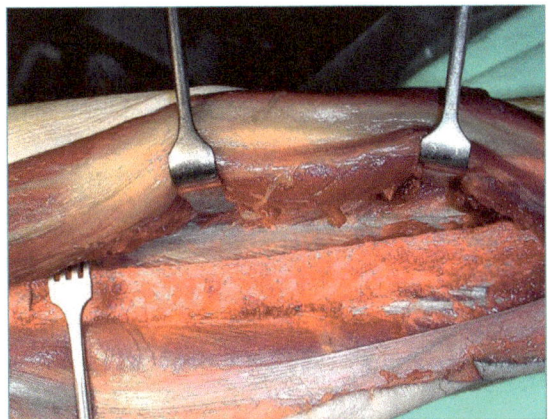

Figure 2.26: In order to restore form and function, a fibula free flap was raised. Picture courtesy of Professor P. Brennan

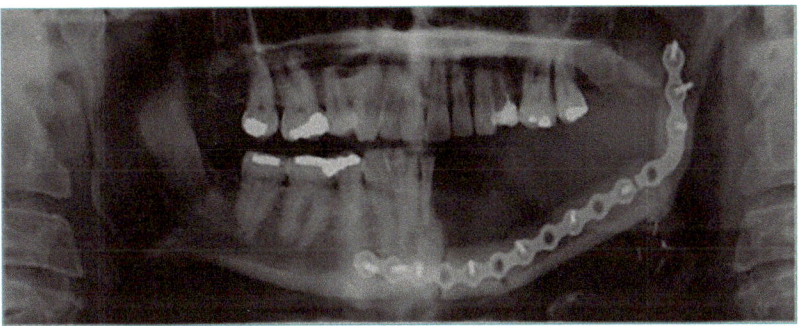

Figure 2.27: This postoperative OPG shows how the fibula bone has been cut or osteotomised to fit the existing profile of the patient. As well as anastomosing the vessels to vessels in the neck, it is secured with plates and screws slightly larger than those normally used in most trauma cases. Picture courtesy of Professor P. Brennan

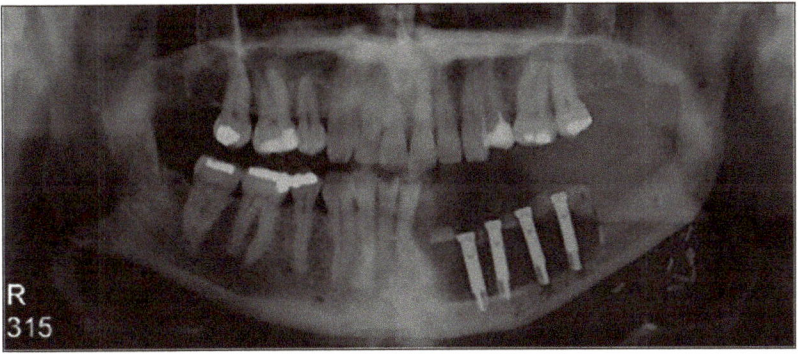

Figure 2.28: Several months later, the patient has gone on to have osseointegrated implants that can be seen on the OPG. Prosthetic teeth can be fitted on these implants to help the patient masticate. Picture courtesy of Professor P. Brennan

34　ORAL AND MAXILLOFACIAL SURGERY

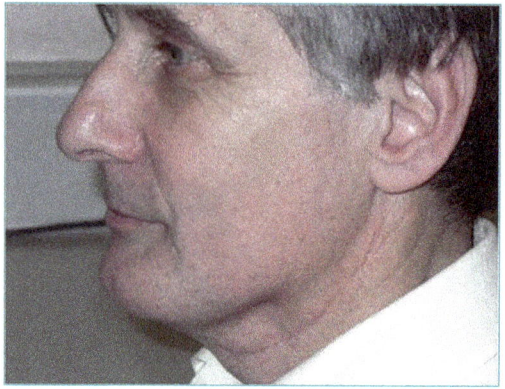
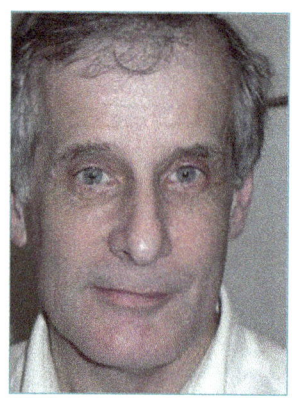

Figures 2.29 & 2.30: These pictures are several months post-surgery. The patient is free from disease, has had a new mandible reconstructed from his fibula and new teeth to eat with. Picture courtesy of Professor P. Brennan

2.5 DENTOALVEOLAR SURGERY

Dentoalveolar surgery is what many would class as 'oral surgery'. Its name indicates that it relates to management of the teeth and the immediate surrounding tissues (gingiva, periodontium and alveolar bone of the jaws) and typically involves the following:

- Exodontia (extraction of teeth, including impacted / orthodontically crowded teeth and removal of root apices for infection)
- Removal of jaw cysts
- Osseointegrated dental implants
- Jaw recontouring work (sulcoplasty/removal of osteotomas, etc.) to facilitate the use of a removable prosthesis for tooth replacement.

The technicalities of dental extraction are beyond the scope of this book but are taught within the dental undergraduate curriculum. Teeth may need to be extracted as a consequence of acquired pathology such as:

1. Dental caries (tooth decay)
2. Periodontal (gum) disease
3. Infection (abscess) or cyst formation secondary to various dental pathologies.

Furthermore, teeth may need to be removed to augment other treatments, such as providing surgical access to a jaw tumour or to aid corrective orthodontic treatment of a dentally 'crowded' jaw.

'Impaction' is the term used to describe where a tooth is unable to fully erupt into the mouth, and is unlikely to do so in the longer term. Not all unerupted teeth are impacted and the patient's age, and thus their expected tooth-eruption dates, aid the diagnosis. Some impacted teeth can simply be monitored by a dentist, but those at risk of, or with, complicating factors such as cyst formation, infection or other pathology may need surgical removal (by drilling away surrounding jaw bone to provide access to, and removal of, the offending tooth/teeth).

Third Molar Surgery

Third molars (also known as 'wisdom teeth') are the teeth most commonly found to be impacted. Those which are partially exposed/erupted in the mouth may lead to pericoronitis – an inflammation or infection of the overlying gum (or operculum) which can trap commensal organisms such as *Peptostreptococci* and *Bacteroides* species.

Early on, this infection may present with discomfort and halitosis and can be treated simply with antiseptic mouth rinses. However, it may progress to facial swelling or even the development of a severe life-threatening neck-space infection causing dysphagia (difficulty swallowing and therefore drooling), odynophagia (painful swallowing) and trismus (reduced mouth opening because of involvement of the masticator/chewing muscles) with accompanying tender swelling of the neck.

There are a number of classification systems used to describe how third molars are impacted, including the Pell and Gregory classification and the Winters classification. Assessment of these teeth for extraction mandates the need for an OPG, which can indicate possible concern about the relationship of the apex of the third molar and the inferior dental nerve (running within the inferior dental canal). Things to look for when deciding whether the tooth is causing impingement of the nerve include:

- Deviation or narrowing of the ID canal
- Loss of the upper tramline of the ID canal
- Darkening/deflection and narrowing of the roots.

Concerns about intimacy of the canal and the root apices may require the use of a CBCT to assess this more comprehensively to decide whether complete extraction of the tooth is required, or whether a coronectomy would be more appropriate.

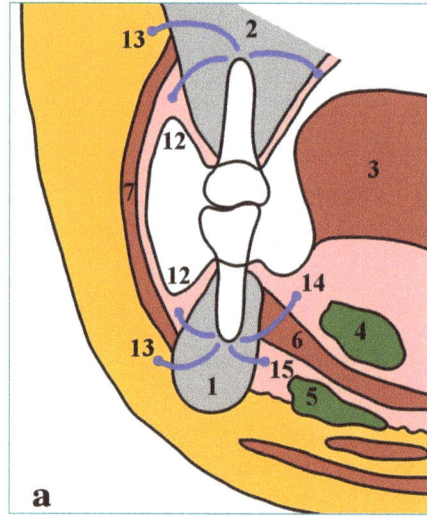
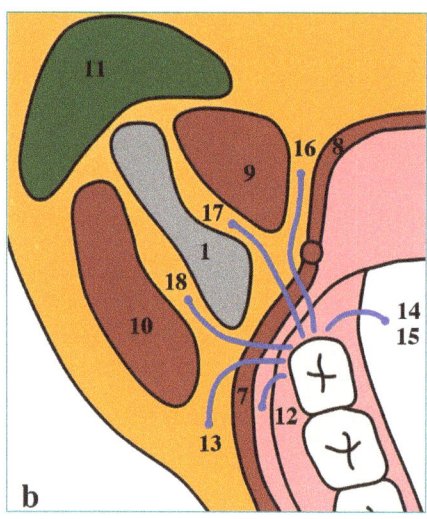

Figure 2.31: (a) Coronal section of cheek and oral cavity, and (b) transverse section at the level of the occlusal plane, to show the routes of spread of dental sepsis.

1. Mandible
2. Maxilla
3. Tongue
4. Sublingual gland
5. Submandibular gland
6. Mylohyoid
7. Buccinator
8. Superior constrictor
9. Medial pterygoid
10. Masseter
11. Parotid gland
12. Buccal sulcus
13. Buccal space
14. Sublingual space
15. Submandibular space
16. Parapharyngeal space
17. Pterygomandibular space
18. Submasseteric space

Impacted Canines

Impacted canines can often present as missing teeth or palatal or buccal lumps/swellings in late childhood/early teens. Maxillary canines should erupt between 11 and 12 years of age. Part of a routine dental assessment of a child involves routinely palpating for their presence around the age of nine years. Removing the deciduous (primary dentition) canine by the age of 10 can in some cases help the adult canine to spontaneously erupt. However, if the adult version does not erupt, it can lead to cyst formation and damage to adjacent teeth (such as resorption of roots of lateral incisors), as well as functional and aesthetic problems.

OMFS or oral surgeons may be called (by an orthodontist) to help by extracting the canine, removing teeth/structures blocking its path, or by drilling through the jaw bone to expose the tooth and attach a small chain with which the orthodontist can gradually pull the tooth into position over a matter of weeks/months (also known as an 'expose and bond' procedure). The impacted canine may be assessed via x-rays, using views from two different angles to locate the precise location of the tooth in 3D. This is often carried out by using an OPG and USO (upper standard occlusal film) or LCPA using the 'SLOB' rule (same lingual opposite buccal). In some cases, a CBCT (3D) scan is indicated to assess whether any root resorption of the permanent dentition is occurring (and to localise the tooth).

Apicectomy

An apicectomy is a procedure sometimes performed when a conventional root canal filling (performed by a dentist) fails because of ongoing periapical infection (around the tip of the tooth root). In an attempt to avoid further infection and loss/removal of tooth tissue, this procedure involves a mucosal flap being raised to allow direct access to the root apex through a window drilled in the jaw bone, followed by placement of some filling material into the root canal in a retrograde manner (i.e. by filling it from the root side of the tooth rather than through the tooth crown itself). This filling material is called 'IRM', but previously amalgam has been used (and can cause tattooing of the overlying mucosa). Success rates for apicectomy vary considerably and are influenced by the calibre of the root canal treatment, size of the apical cyst and access considerations.

We'll revisit this in the next chapter when we look at cysts of the jaw.

Implants

Attempts to replace missing teeth are reported as far back as 600BC. Ever since the 1960s there has been huge progression in the use of dental implants, to the point that oral and maxillofacial surgeons commonly place osseointegrated titanium dental implant fixtures. This can be done as part of major reconstructions (for example, placing implants into a jaw reconstructed with a fibular free flap). Implants can also be placed in isolation (with or without the additional use of bone graft material) when replacing teeth for simpler functional and aesthetic reasons (usually in conjunction with a restorative dentist who deals with the non-surgical aspects).

There is a growing interest in how implants can be used. As maxillofacial surgeons we can use 'dental' implants to aid in the rehabilitation of patients who may require replacement of an eye or an ear (because of loss associated with cancer or trauma). You may also hear of zygomatic implants being used where conventional dental implants are not practical, again to aid restoration of function with a fixed bridge or denture.

2.6 CLEFT LIP AND PALATE

Cleft lip and palate is the most common congenital craniofacial deformity and occurs in between one in 700 and one in 1,000 births. Cleft lip, with or without cleft palate, and isolated cleft palate are considered two very separate clinical entities. Clefts occur when the structures of the lip or palate fail to fuse during development in the womb. This failure to fuse causes a gap (or 'cleft') in the tissues. Alongside obvious aesthetic issues, this can result in problems with regards to feeding, speech and hearing, as well as tooth development and maxillary jaw growth.

While a number of syndromes are associated with cleft lip and palate, and cleft palate, the pathogenesis is multifactorial. The majority of cleft-lip-and-palate

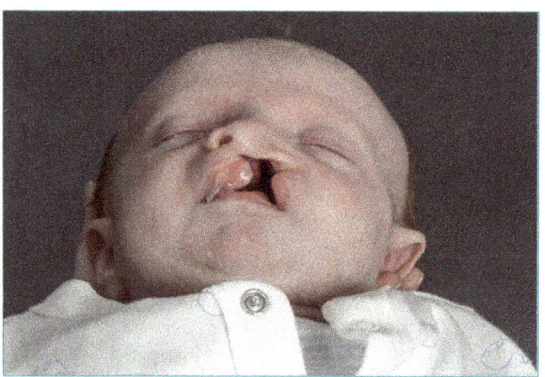

Figure 2.32: Complete cleft lip and palate. Notice the incomplete lip seal, nasal distortion and extension into the nasal cavity. Picture courtesy of Miss Victoria Beale

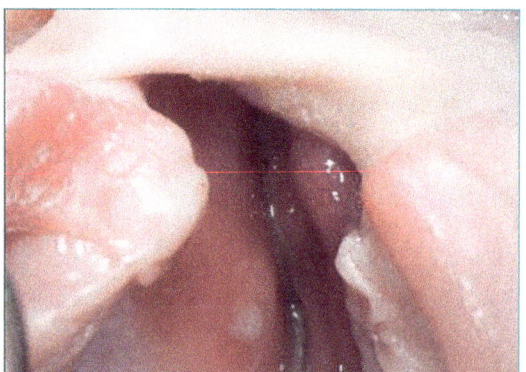

Figure 2.33: Intra-oral view of complete cleft palate on the same child – left side. You can appreciate the challenges this will present in a new-born and with feeding, as there is an incomplete oral-cavity seal which extends from the alveolar crest anteriorly onto the soft palate. Picture courtesy of Miss Victoria Beale

cases are isolated non-syndromic birth defects; however, a small proportion are part of a syndrome such as hemifacial microsomia. Cleft lip alone accounts for around 25% of cleft-lip-and-palate cases. Cleft palate can present with a varying range of severity from partial to complete clefting of the soft and hard palate. (Unlike cleft lip and palate, isolated cleft palate has a far greater association with rare syndromes such as Van der Woude syndrome, Stickler syndrome and DiGeorge syndrome.)

Assessment

Historical improvements in antenatal ultrasound mean that cleft lip and palate can now be diagnosed as early as 12-weeks gestation, but sensitivity increases from week 20 onwards. Although antenatal diagnosis is most common, ultrasound is poorly sensitive in identifying an isolated cleft palate. Furthermore, a significant proportion of cleft lip and palate is still diagnosed at birth as part of the new-born baby assessment.

Management

The management of cleft lip and palate is multidisciplinary, requiring the input of cleft surgeons, otologists, paediatricians, orthodontists, speech and language therapists, and specialist nurses. From the surgeon's point of view, surgery is done throughout the child and young adult's lifespan and involves meticulous management of skin, mucosa, musculature and bone in order to achieve anatomical harmony (see table below).

Age	Treatment
3–4 months	Cleft lip repair
8–15 months (typically at 6–9 months in the UK)	Cleft palate repair
6–13 years	Alveolar bone grafting followed by orthodontics
12–21 years	Orthognathic surgery
	Rhinoplasty
	Revisional surgery (e.g. pharyngoplasty)

Table: Timing of surgical procedures in cleft patients

New-borns often have a capacity to compensate for their cleft whilst suckling and their swallowing is otherwise normal, but sometimes modified feeding devices are needed in the first few months. Nevertheless, cleft lip can make a lip seal difficult: lip repair is performed at approximately three months of age and is based upon some key principles:

1. Excision of poor-quality tissues at the margins of the cleft
2. Approximate the lip segments whilst preserving natural landmarks (e.g. cupid's bow)
3. Place scars along natural lines to try to make them as inconspicuous as possible
4. Restore symmetry to the lip, nostril margins and alar bases
5. Account for vermillion height deficiency in the cleft side by recruiting tissue from the lateral lip.

Repair of the cleft palate from eight months onwards is principally for the development of future intelligible speech (and avoiding air rushing through the palate and out of the nose, known as hyper-nasal speech). The aims of a functional palatal repair are as follows:

1. Achieving normal, intelligible speech
2. To aid feeding
3. To prevent restriction of maxillary growth.

Palatal muscles are dissected from their tethered abnormal muscle insertions into the nasal and oral mucosa. Most importantly, repositioning the levator veli palatini muscle recreates the 'levator sling', a continuous band of muscle across the soft palate which partly recreates the velopharyngeal sphincter (allowing control of the desired airflow through the mouth or nose into and out of the pharynx, and therefore control of the nasality of speech). Velopharyngeal insufficiency presents with hyper-nasal speech and abnormal findings on videofluoroscopy and nasoendoscopy.

For speech problems that cannot be managed by speech therapy alone, pharyngeal obturators or further surgery to restrict nasal air escape may be needed (such as pharyngoplasty).

Alveolar bone grafting is needed when the cleft involves the tooth-bearing bone, without which a persistent oronasal fistula (connection between the mouth and nose with leakage of fluids between) will result.

Subsequent and Ongoing Care

Throughout childhood, the cleft MDT work to promote effective management on speech, feeding, hearing, growth and the treatment of other associated congenital disorders (if present). Cleft patients may have complex physical and mental needs throughout their adult lives as well, requiring a very holistic approach to their care. In early adulthood, functional and aesthetic problems of the jaws and nose require orthognathic surgery (sometimes involving distraction osteogenesis) to address the hypoplastic maxilla (retrusive upper jaw) and septorhinoplasty (possibly multiple nasal surgeries) for the associated complex nasal deformity.

2.7 DENTAL TRAUMA

One of the things you will often be asked about managing is dental trauma, which is beyond the scope of this textbook; but needless to say, confidence in assessing the dentition as an OMFS team member is mandatory, as well as knowing when you can offer advice, when you need to splint teeth and when you need to perform an urgent extraction (if there is a potential airway risk). The Dental Trauma Guideline website (https://dentaltraumaguide.org/) is a useful resource to identify what you should do. It provides advice to give patients and directs colleagues to evidence-based practice on best management.

Depending upon your local resources, you may be able to refer to and access maxillofacial prosthetic scientists (through the maxillofacial unit) who can help with custom-made blow-down splints to manage trauma where splinting using conventional composite and wire is impractical or challenging.

CHAPTER 3: THE JAWS

3.1 ANATOMY AND EMBRYOLOGY

By the fifth week of intra-uterine development, the face consists of five facial prominences:

- Fronto-nasal prominence
- Paired maxillary prominences
- Paired mandibular prominences.

Between weeks five and eight of intra-uterine development, a number of these processes fuse. Abnormalities in this process can result in various clefts including a laterally deflected nose, cleft lip and/or palate, as we discussed in the previous chapter.

Together, the mandible and maxilla form the framework of the oral cavity, thereby playing a crucial role in mastication, swallowing and speech. It would be a good starting point before reading this chapter to remind yourself of the bony anatomy of the maxilla and mandible (including the inferior alveolar nerve passing into the mandible at the mandibular foramen and exiting at the mental foramen, where it provides sensation to the lower lip and chin), the temporomandibular joint (TMJ) (including the condyle, disc and glenoid fossa in the temporal bone) and the muscles of mastication (including masseter, temporalis, medial pterygoid and lateral pterygoid). These muscles of mastication are innervated by the trigeminal nerve. In contrast, the muscles of facial expression are innervated by the facial nerve.

3.2 FRACTURES OF THE MANDIBLE AND MIDFACE

3.2.1 MANDIBULAR FRACTURES

Facial trauma is very common and, given its location, the mandible often bears the brunt of such force. As oral and maxillofacial surgeons, we see a myriad of facial injuries but will always have a high suspicion for mandibular trauma. As with all fractures, a focused history and examination are crucial and further investigations, such as imaging, should seek to confirm the precise location and orientation of any fracture and assess the degree of displacement (if any) of the bony fragments. A mandible fracture may present in a clinically obvious way but sometimes the signs are more subtle, especially with non-displaced fractures.

On examination, you might see a clearly visible deformity of the jaw; pain and swelling around the jaw; teeth that are out of line and don't meet correctly (altered occlusion); a gingival tear and bleeding within the oral cavity; and possibly numbness (paraesthesia) of the lip and chin due to damage to the inferior alveolar nerve.

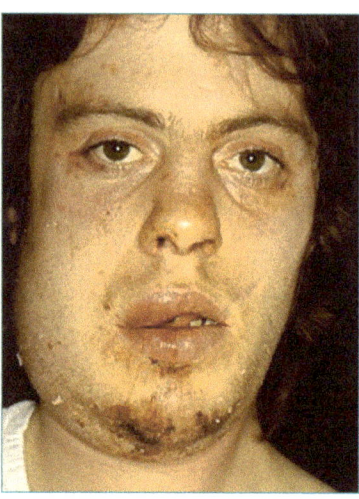

Figure 3.1: This gentleman has been assaulted. He has a right-sided facial swelling and reports a change in feeling to his lower lip. Picture courtesy of Mr. Graham Bounds

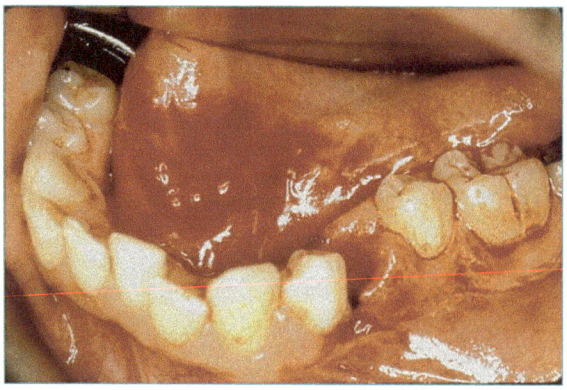

Figure 3.2: Intra-oral examination of a potential fractured mandible can show gingival tears, movement of teeth from their sockets, bleeding and haematoma formation. Picture courtesy of Mr. Graham Bounds

Any of the above should prompt plain film radiography in the first instance, or if part of a major trauma ('polytrauma'), a head-to-toe CT scan. For mandible fractures alone, an orthopantomogram (OPG) in combination with a PA (postero-anterior) mandible plain film is all that's needed. In essence, the OPG 'flattens' out the jaw from a 'U' shape to provide a 2D image and the PA mandible provides a back-to-front look at the mandible, which is particularly useful for assessing fracture displacement.

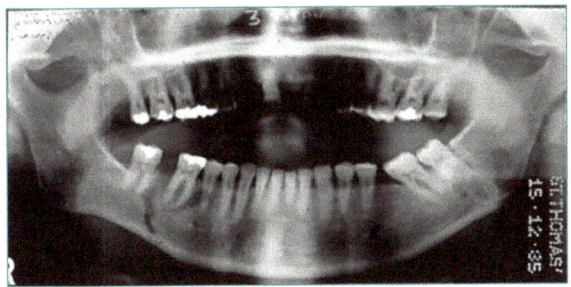

Figure 3.3: This is an OPG. Notice how it flattens out the jaw and is useful for assessment of the TMJ, dental pathology and also fractures. Here, a fracture of the right body and left angle can be seen. Picture courtesy of Mr. Graham Bounds

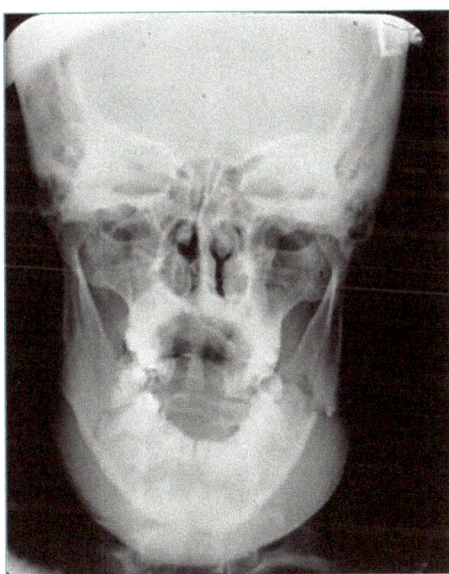

Figure 3.4: This PA (postero-anterior) mandibular plain film provides a back-to-front look at the mandible. This, together with an OPG, is the first-line investigation for a fractured mandible. Picture courtesy of Mr. Graham Bounds

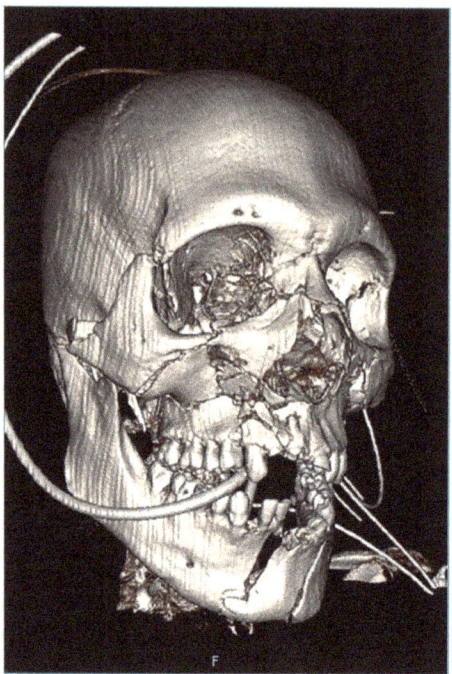

Figure 3.5: This is a 3D reformat of a patient with extensive facial injuries sustained after jumping from a bridge. This gives you an immediate idea of the extent of the injuries here, which include fractures to mandible, maxilla and nasal and zygomatic complexes bilaterally. Picture courtesy of Miss Elizabeth Yeung

Management

To consider the management and surgical treatment of mandibular fractures, one must first recap the bony anatomy of the mandible and the separate regions we define. The mandible is described as having a condyle, coronoid process, ascending ramus, angle, body, parasymphysis and symphysis. As the mandible is a 'U' shape, trauma to one side of the jaw will often cause contralateral injury (i.e. a double fracture). One way of thinking about this is to visualise the breaking of a 'polo mint', which would break into two sections.

As you see more of these, you will come to appreciate patterns of injury that are very common – for example, an angle fracture with a contralateral condyle fracture. Or a 'Guardsman' fracture – a bilateral fracture of the condyles and symphysis, named so due to the history of guardsmen collapsing during duty, falling forwards onto their jaw and thus causing this common fracture pattern.

You may also hear fractures described as 'favourable' or 'unfavourable'; simply put, this describes the orientation of the fracture in relation to the pull of the surrounding musculature. A fracture that is supported and held in place by the pull of a group of muscles is less likely to be displaced and may lend itself to more conservative (i.e. non-operative) treatment.

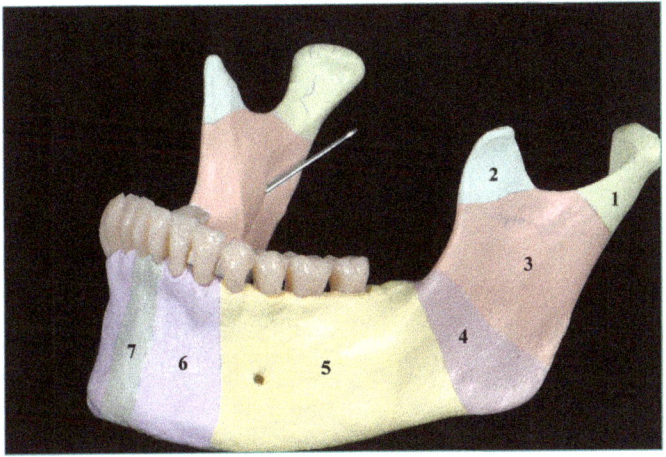

Figure 3.6: Anatomy of the mandible with regard to the description of a fracture site (silver pin on right side indicating path of ID nerve entering mandibular foramen).

1. Condyle
2. Coronoid process
3. Ramus
4. Angle
5. Body
6. Parasymphysis
7. Symphysis

Treatment of a fractured mandible is to promote improved pain, restoration of function and aesthetics alongside promotion of healing.

When we talk about surgical management of a mandible fracture, we are asking the question: 'do we need to stabilise the jaw, or will the fracture heal on its own?' If the fracture is non-displaced and favourable with a co-operative patient, it's reasonable to trial a period of conservative treatment and review the patient after one week.

On the other hand, if the fracture is going to move then the bone won't heal, so we would need to reduce and stabilise the bony fragments. We can do this via a 'closed reduction', where we don't surgically expose the fracture, but we use the teeth or bone to guide the fracture into place and hold it securely in position with brackets and wires around the teeth. Alternatively, we may need to surgically open the fracture site, reduce the bony fragments and fix them in the correct anatomical position using small but very strong titanium plates and screws. This is called 'open reduction, internal fixation' (ORIF).

The above principles are applied in general to most mandible fractures, with the exception of certain sub-sites, such as the mandibular condyle, which have their own specific treatment and more complex management algorithms due

48   ORAL AND MAXILLOFACIAL SURGERY

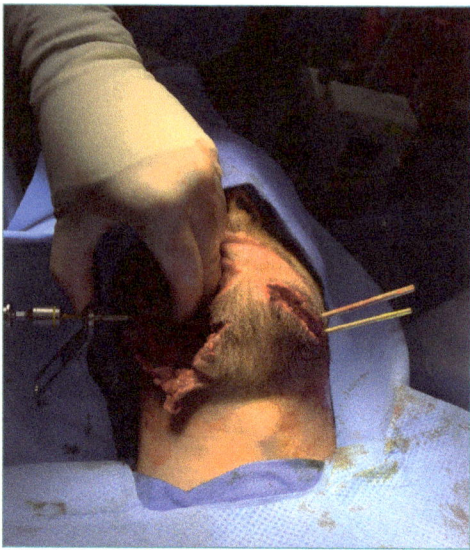

Figure 3.7: The patient required open reduction internal fixation of the mandible. Where possible, we try to do all of this from inside the oral cavity. In some instances, such as this, we have to approach the fracture from an extra-oral route. Picture courtesy of Lieutenant Colonel Johno Breeze

to their proximity to key anatomical structures such as the facial nerve and the parotid gland.

3.2.2 MIDFACE FRACTURES

The midface is a complex structure derived from the union of a number of bones. The largest bone of the midface is the maxilla, which provides support to the tooth-bearing structures, sinuses, globes and muscles of facial expression.

1. Maxillary Fractures

Because the maxilla has several anatomical functions, the presentation of these fractures can be varied – from no clinical signs but with a subtle fracture on imaging, to gross comminution ('shattering' into multiple pieces) and displacement. Such signs you may see include: movement of teeth and an altered occlusion; mobility of the bone; potential for significant bleeding; and involvement of the orbits and zygomatic bone (discussed below).

Classification

Midface fractures are commonly classified according to Le Fort patterns. This eponymous classification is named after René Le Fort, a French surgeon who spent his spare time hitting cadaveric skulls with clubs and cannon balls, and in doing so identified three key fracture patterns resulting from blunt-force trauma. The midface fractures occurred in specific patterns because of the facial buttresses (three horizontal and three vertical) that dictate the

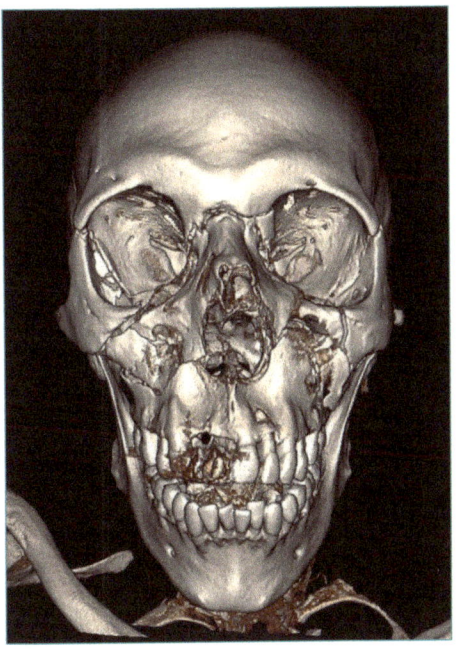

Figure 3.8: A patient with a fractured maxilla can often present with epistaxis, an elongated face and an anterior open bite. This is where they are biting on their back teeth, but their front teeth are wide apart. This is because the maxilla is pushed backwards, 'jacking open' their occlusion. Picture courtesy of Mr. Graham Bounds

distribution of forces through the bone. These buttresses are strong and denser vertical and horizontal columns of bone that provide form and functional strength to the midface.

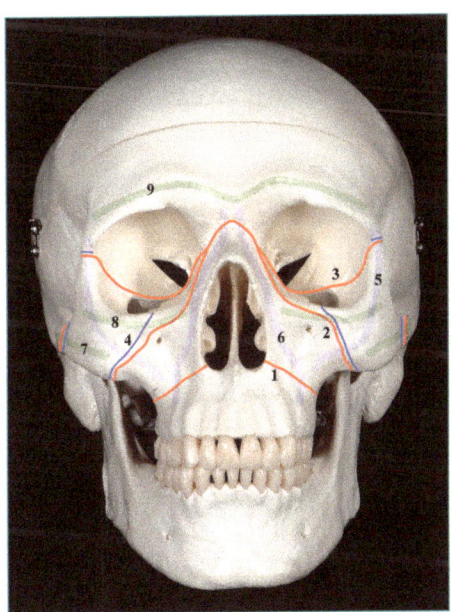

Figure 3.9: Midface buttresses and fracture patterns displayed on a skull.

1. *Le Fort I fracture*
2. *Le Fort II fracture*
3. *Le Fort III fracture*
4. *Zygomatic complex fracture*
5. *Zygomatic vertical buttress*
6. *Nasofrontal vertical buttress*
7. *Zygomatic arch horizontal buttress*
8. *Infraorbital horizontal buttress*
9. *Supraorbital horizontal buttress*

Midfacial fractures can be categorised as follows:	
Dentoalveolar	A fracture involving only the dentoalveolar part of the maxilla (or mandible).
Le Fort I	Horizontal fracture line separating palate from maxillary complex, running just above floor of nasal cavity (Figure 3.9).
Le Fort II	Horizontal fracture line involving anterolateral walls of maxillary sinuses and crossing bridge of nose superiorly ('pyramidal') (Figure 3.9).
Le Fort III ('craniofacial dysjunction')	High horizontal fracture through nasofrontal buttress (involving cribriform plate, therefore mechanical and infection risk to olfactory nerves and other contents of anterior cranial fossa), orbital floors and zygomatico-frontal sutures laterally (Figure 3.9).
Nasal and naso-orbito-ethmoidal (NOE) complex fractures	Fracture pattern depends on the direction and magnitude of force. A horizontal blow may cause only a lateral shift of the nasal bones, whereas a frontal blow is more likely to result in buckling of the septum and ethmoidal involvement as the septum is driven posteriorly. NOE fractures are associated with additional frontal or anterior cranial fossa fractures and, like Le Fort III injuries, you should maintain a high suspicion for intracranial injury.
Zygomatic arch and zygomatic complex	Both may lead to flattening of the malar prominence, which can be very pronounced with a fracture of the zygomatic complex. With a zygomatic complex fracture, posterior displacement can interrupt the orbital floor, leading to ocular complications (see section 6.4 on orbital fractures) (Figure 3.9).

Table: The Le Fort classification

Management

It is commonly accepted that Le Fort fractures should be operated on within 10–14 days of injury, after initial swelling has reduced (or very soon after the injury, before any significant swelling occurs), as soft-tissue swelling can make anatomical repositioning of fracture segments more difficult. Depending on the type of fracture, we can access these in the form of intra-oral incisions, lower eyelid incisions or via a scalp-based coronal flap (in order to reduce any cosmetic surgical scarring to the face). Surgery will take the form of ORIF, with titanium miniplates and screws. The primary aim of midfacial surgery will be to restore the continuity of bone by strengthening the previously mentioned facial buttresses.

AN ILLUSTRATED GUIDE 51

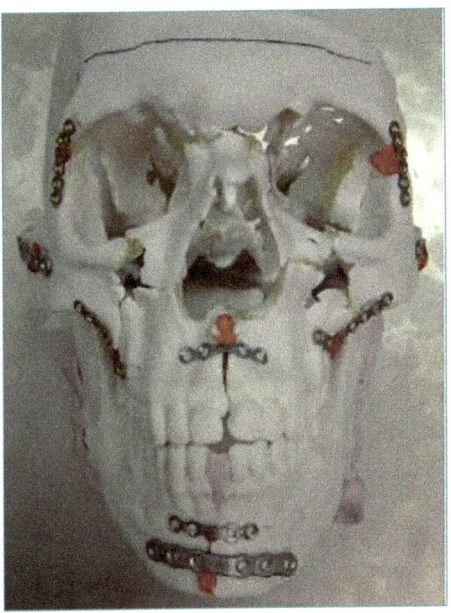

Figure 3.10: 3D-printed model with fracture reduction planned in the lab of a pan-facial case with plates pre-bent to aid intra-operative fixation. Picture courtesy of Mr. Jason Watson

This type of extensive surgery can be planned and executed with the use of 3D-printed models and pre-bent plates to aid reduction and promote accuracy of fixation. Ask your local maxillofacial unit if they have an onsite printing facility for this purpose.

2. Zygomatic Complex Fractures

The zygomatic bone, or zygoma, provides width and profile to the face. It articulates with the frontal bone above, the maxilla below and, via its 'arch', with the temporal bone. It also forms a significant portion of the lateral wall of the orbit.

As expected, injuries to the zygoma are not uncommon, due to its prominent position on the lateral part of the face. In general, we group zygomatic fractures into more simple 'zygomatic-arch fractures' and 'tripod' (better described as 'quadripod' or 'zygomatic complex') fractures, whereby the zygoma can fracture at three points of union with nearby facial bones, which displaces the entire body of the zygoma (or zygomatic complex). The term 'tripod' is something of a misnomer because there are actually four key points of fracture: lateral orbit, zygomaticomaxillary buttress, arch of zygoma and the orbital floor. As we will discuss in Chapter 6, the orbital-floor component can cause numerous eye signs and symptoms.

52 ORAL AND MAXILLOFACIAL SURGERY

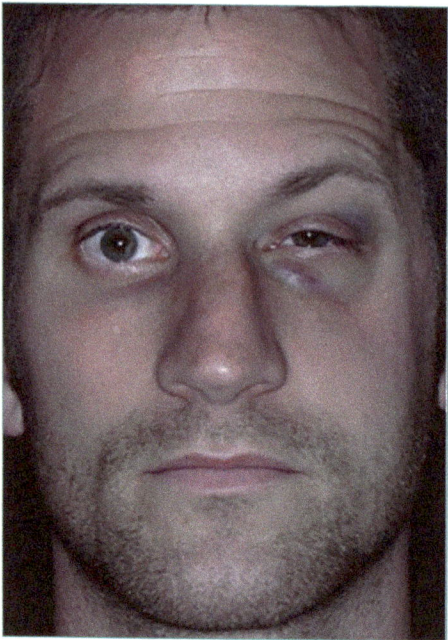

Figure 3.11: The zygoma provides width to the face. Here you can see the flattening of the left cheekbone or zygoma. This can also cause peri-orbital ecchymosis, subconjunctival haemorrhage and infra-orbital sensory loss. Picture courtesy of Mr. Graham Bounds

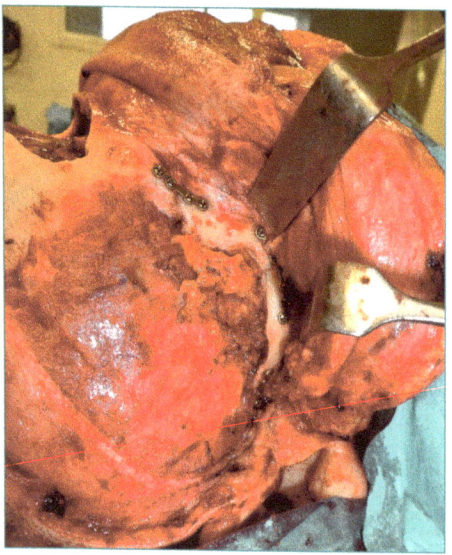

Figure 3.12: Here you can see the zygoma has fractured at the lateral orbital wall, called the 'zygomatico-frontal suture', and on the arch itself. It has been fixed with miniplates and screws via a coronal approach. This is not always required, as we can usually approach the zygoma with inconspicuous incisions. Picture courtesy of Mr. Madan Ethunandan

When you examine a patient with a zygomatic fracture, you might see a visible flattening of the cheekbone, decreased mouth opening (if a fractured zygomatic arch is impinging the coronoid process of the mandible where the temporalis muscle attaches); and/or orbital involvement. The patient may complain of numbness of the cheek due to infra-orbital nerve involvement.

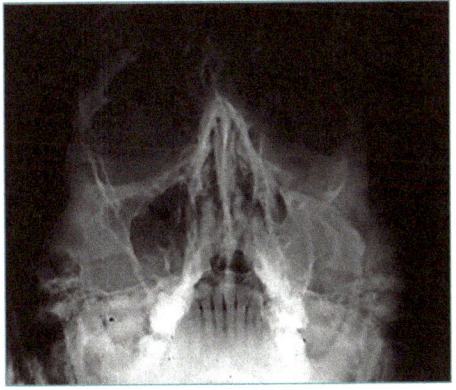

Figure 3.13: This occipitomental radiograph indicated a left zygoma fracture. Again, when assessing such x-rays, it is useful to look for symmetry, or in this case asymmetry. Picture courtesy of Mr. Graham Bounds

Eye signs and symptoms may include swelling, subconjunctival haemorrhage, double vision (diplopia) and reduced eye movement (particularly in the upward gaze).

Surgery is performed when there is an aesthetic or functional deformity. Again, we normally wait 10–14 days to allow the swelling to settle and for additional injuries such as orbital-floor/wall defects to manifest and be assessed accordingly. For isolated zygomatic arch fractures, these can be simply 'lifted' back into place via a Gilles approach, as shown in Figure 3.14, to restore normal facial contour.

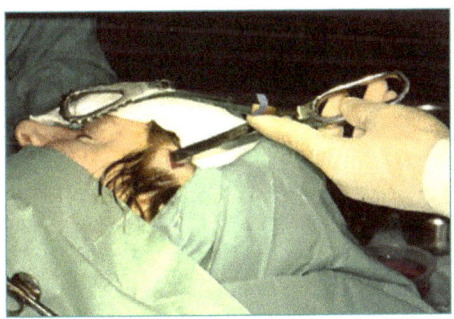

Figure 3.14: As we have highlighted throughout this book, oral and maxillofacial surgeons attempt to minimise facial deformity as best as possible. Here the zygoma is lifted into the correct position through an incision, which is placed in the hair to hide it. Picture courtesy of Mr. Graham Bounds

3.3 JAW DEFORMITY

Orthognathic Surgery

Facial deformity occurs as a consequence of abnormal skeletal, soft tissue and dental relationships in the horizontal, transverse or vertical planes. Orthognathic surgery is the sub-speciality interest area of OMFS concerned with correcting such deformities. More recently, orthognathic surgery is also being performed as a highly effective treatment for obstructive sleep apnoea, as forward movement of the jaws can improve airflow through the naso- and oropharynx.

Some facial deformities are associated with syndromic conditions, sometimes with an underlying genetic aetiology. However, more often the deformity will be multifactorial, due to an abnormality of skeletal bone growth, functional muscle attachments and environmental influences. We see this commonly in the cleft-palate patient who has a retrusive maxilla (and a Class 3 occlusion as a result).

When we assess a patient with a facial skeletal discrepancy who is requesting treatment, we are primarily concerned with improving their function. This may help with the patient's bite and chewing, or even speech and swallowing. Improving function is achieved via restoring the 'normal' form and relationship of the facial skeleton and soft tissues. Clearly this will have an impact on the facial profile, and is a consideration, but this is not the primary aim of orthognathic surgery.

3.3.1 ASSESSMENT

A thorough history and clinical assessment are performed for all orthognathic patients. This must include existing functional issues, any TMJ complaints and a detailed discussion of the patient's ideas and expectations. Usually, a pre-designed proforma will be used to ensure all facial measurements are recorded accurately. It is outside the scope of this book to detail the terminology and examination of a facial deformity patient. However, this allows for an extensive assessment of the patient against 'normal' parameters, from which a treatment plan can be created in conjunction with an orthodontist (dental specialist) and OMFS laboratory staff.

You will be familiar with the concept of a Class 1, Class 2 and Class 3 occlusion which we'll discuss further in the next chapter. It may be helpful to you to revisit these concepts with respect to the facial profile before reading on.

3.3.2 EXAMINATION

Assessing a facial deformity is often quite challenging. You should now be aware that we divide the face into 'thirds' and that most often we are concerned with the 'middle third' (i.e. the maxilla) and the 'lower third' (i.e. the mandible) when considering performing surgery to these bones.

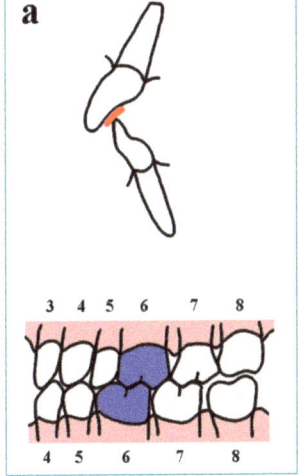
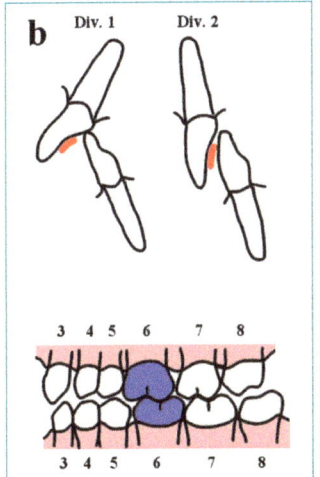
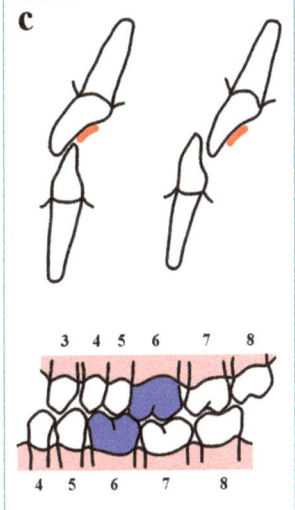

Figure 3.15: Classifications of dental occlusion based upon central incisor and first molar relationships:
  a) Class I
  b) Class II (Division 1 and Division 2)
  c) Class III

It might sound simple, but the goal of examination is to determine the specific facial component (bone, soft tissue or both) contributing to the deformity – i.e. is the middle third overdeveloped or is the lower third underdeveloped and vice versa. A key component of our decision is the relationship of the top and bottom teeth. We describe this according to how the incisors meet. A Class I relationship, where the upper incisors are 2–4mm in front of the lower incisors, is considered 'normal'. In a Class II relationship, the upper incisors are greater than 4mm in front of the lowers; and in a Class III relationship, the lower jaw protrudes so that the lower incisors are in front of the upper incisors.

56 ORAL AND MAXILLOFACIAL SURGERY

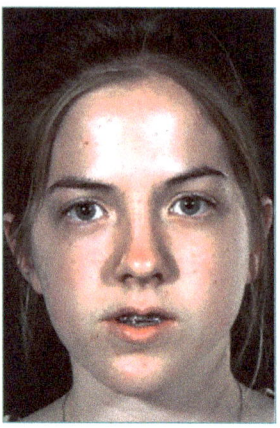

Figure 3.16: Looking at this young lady from 'front on', it looks very much like her chin is pointing more to the right. Picture courtesy of Mr. Andrew Sidebottom

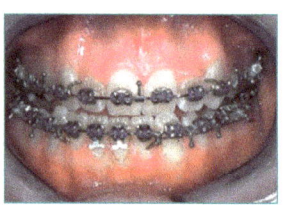

Figure 3.17: As you can see, her top-teeth (jaw) midline is not coincident with the lower-teeth (jaw) midline. Picture courtesy of Mr. Andrew Sidebottom

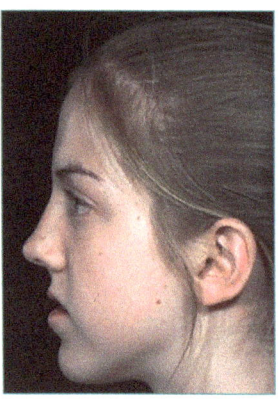

Figure 3.18: From the side, it looks like the lower jaw is slightly in front of the upper jaw. This would be considered a Class III skeletal pattern or jaw relationship. Picture courtesy of Mr. Andrew Sidebottom

3.3.3 TREATMENT

Treatment for skeletal discrepancies is an entire treatment pathway not one discreet surgical procedure and involves joint care with both OMFS surgeons and orthodontists. At the initial assessment, they will use photographs, impressions of the teeth and radiographs to detail the patient's baseline skeletal and soft-tissue relationship.

Conventional treatment commences with orthodontic treatment (braces) for several months, in preparation for surgery followed by post-surgical orthodontics – all taking up to two years or more. This is known as dental decompensation in preparation for surgery, and can result in exacerbating the existing malocclusion in preparation for surgery. However, there is an increasing interest in a 'surgery-first' orthognathic approach, where the osteotomy is done first, and then braces used to finish aligning and co-ordinating the arches.

Surgical Treatment for Facial Deformity

Having considered the above, the goal of surgery is to break the jaw bones in a controlled and careful way, and then to move them into a more functionally favourable position (known as an 'osteotomy'). Having done this, we then fix the bones in their new position with titanium plates and screws – the same ones we use for facial trauma, as mentioned before. There are countless surgical techniques and fixation devices used to achieve this goal. Commonly, surgery to the mandible is termed a 'bilateral sagittal split osteotomy' (so-called because of the orientation of the cut through the ramus of the mandible). Surgery to the maxilla is termed a 'Le Fort I osteotomy' (as the fracture created is similar to the fracture pattern described earlier). These procedures are either performed in isolation or together to achieve a greater degree of dental and bony movement. When performed together, the procedure is termed a 'bimaxillary osteotomy' – a historical term from when the jaws were termed the 'upper and lower maxillae'.

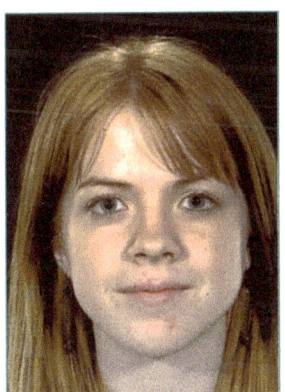 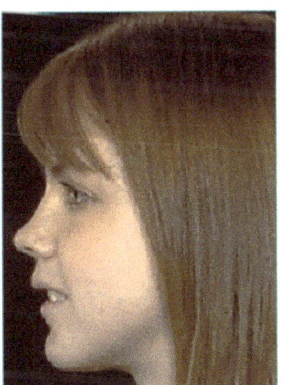

Figures 3.19 & 3.20: This young lady underwent a condylar shave to treat condylar hyperplasia and a bimaxillary osteotomy to move both jaws. As you can see, her chin is now in the midline and her lower jaw is behind her upper jaw. Pictures courtesy of Mr. Andrew Sidebottom

Additional Procedures

Additional surgery may include genioplasty to reshape the chin, or palatal expansion surgery to widen the upper jaw. Furthermore, movement of the jaws can affect the appearance of the nose and sometimes even a second-stage rhinoplasty is performed.

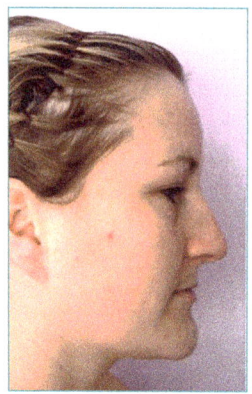
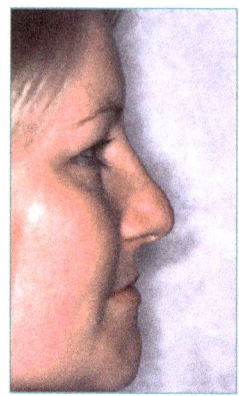

Figures 3.21 & 3.22. This lady underwent a reduction genioplasty and rhinoplasty. Note that you can see her chin in the second photo in more in line with her upper jaw. Pictures courtesy of Mr Andrew Sidebottom.

3.3.4 DISTRACTION OSTEOGENESIS

An alternative to moving bones and fixing them in one procedure is 'distraction osteogenesis'. This was described by the orthopaedic surgeon Ilizarov, who proposed the technique after treating patients with lower bony-limb injuries after the Second World War. In maxillofacial applications, we break the bones (undertake corticotomy) and insert a distracting device to slowly (0.5–1mm per day) pull them apart, and wait for the callus to form as we distract. Such an approach is useful in paediatric syndromic patients with gross deformities not amenable to a single-stage procedure. It involves three stages after the corticotomy:

1. Latent phase (can vary from 1–3 days)
2. Distraction phase (at a rate of 0.5–1mm a day until the planned movement is achieved)
3. Consolidation phase to allow callus maturation and bony healing to occur.

The main advantage of distraction osteogenesis is that, because of the slower nature of movement achieved, the soft tissues also stretch to accommodate.

3.4 THE TEMPOROMANDIBULAR JOINT (TMJ)

3.4.1 ANATOMY

The TMJ is a complex region of the facial skeleton. It is comprised of the condylar head of the mandible, the glenoid fossa at the base of the skull, a cartilaginous intra-articular disc separating an upper and lower compartment, each filled with synovial fluid, surrounded by an overlying joint capsule and influenced by muscles of mastication. Pain and dysfunction of the TMJ is now thought to be a multifactorial problem, sometimes with a strong contributing psychological component. It is a common clinical complaint seen frequently by dentists, who can refer onwards to OMFS surgeons following a period of non-surgical management.

3.4.2 EXAMINING THE TMJ

When examining the TMJ, we are assessing the gross function of the joint to open and close the mouth, and then also signs on the teeth that may be causing or exacerbating a TMJ problem. We will ask the patient to open and close their mouth (and in doing so formally record their maximal incisal opening), looking for equal and symmetrical movement and assessing whether they have an adequate degree of mouth opening. We can then examine the teeth, palpate the TMJ for pain and crepitus, and palpate the muscles of mastication (masseter, temporalis, lateral and medial pterygoids).

For example, a patient who grinds their teeth can cause trauma to the TMJ as a result, due to overworked muscle pulling causing strain on the joint. They may show signs of tooth wear and/or masseteric hypertrophy. There may be evidence of linea alba or scalloping of the tongue on intra-oral examination. A baseline OPG radiograph will screen for any obvious TMJ bony abnormality, and can be supported by a CT scan to support planned intervention. Very rarely an MRI may be required, depending on the severity and nature of the TMJ dysfunction.

3.4.3 TEMPOROMANDIBULAR JOINT DISORDER (TMJD)

Although TMJD has been through several incarnations of terminology and classifications, in essence it describes a condition with one or several symptoms of jaw dysfunction – specifically pain, trismus (reduced mouth opening of less than 30mm in an adult), restricted lateral mandibular movement, joint locking and crepitus (or 'clicking'). It is a common condition and affects up to 50% of the population at some point in their lifetimes. We often see dental students who present to us with this problem, and it can be associated with stress or even pending exams. As alluded to, such cases are often complex and multifactorial in nature. Whilst the distinction is not always clear, for treatment purposes it is useful to think of TMJD as being articular (to do with the joint itself) or non-articular (due to overworked muscles of mastication).

Clicking jaw joints, with no pain, do not require any surgical intervention and can be managed in primary care by a general dentist or GP.

Management

The treatment of TMJD is tailored to the underlying cause. Pain and dysfunction originating from a non-articular cause are often myofascial (soft tissue) in origin and rarely require surgical intervention. Identification and subsequent cessation of any parafunctional habits such as pen-lid chewing or nail-biting can aid management. Adjuncts such as a bite guard may help night-time grinding, and local measures can ease muscular pain (such as a hot compress, regular NSAIDS in the form of gel, jaw physiotherapy and a soft diet). Pain that is chronic in nature may benefit from tricyclic antidepressant medication such as nortriptyline or amitriptyline.

Articular disease is associated with an abnormality of the joint itself. Whilst the majority of cases are idiopathic, history of previous mandibular trauma, or joint diseases such as septic arthritis, osteoarthritis or rheumatoid arthritis can point towards a definitive organic diagnosis.

Options for surgical intervention include arthrocentesis (washout of the joint to reduce inflammation), arthroscopy (to wash out and inspect the joint using a small camera, and sometimes minimally operate on the joint) and lastly, open joint surgery. A degenerative condition of the TMJ that is refractory to conservative treatment may eventually require replacement of the joint. In this instance, the joint is exposed surgically and a joint prosthesis implanted to restore function, either with unilateral or bilateral surgery. This surgery is technically very challenging – and the facial nerve is intimately related to the TMJ, too!

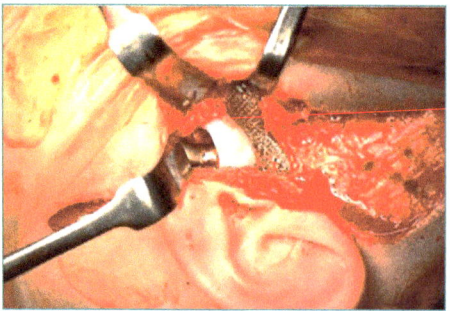

Figure 3.23: This is an intra-operative picture of a TMJ replacement. An incision is hidden in a crease in front of the ear. Great care is taken to find access to the joint without compromising the facial nerve or its branches. Picture courtesy of Mr. Andrew Sidebottom

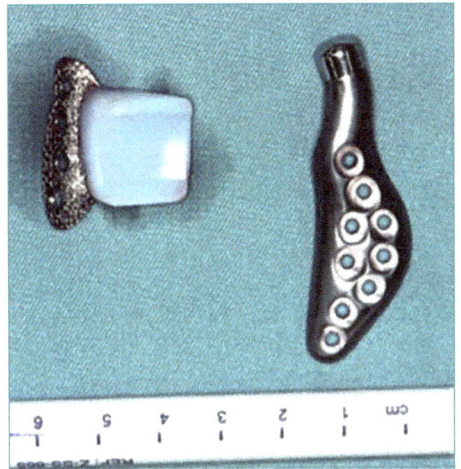

Figure 3.24: This is a prosthetic mandibular condyle (right side of picture) and glenoid fossa (left side of picture). Picture courtesy of Mr. Andrew Sidebottom

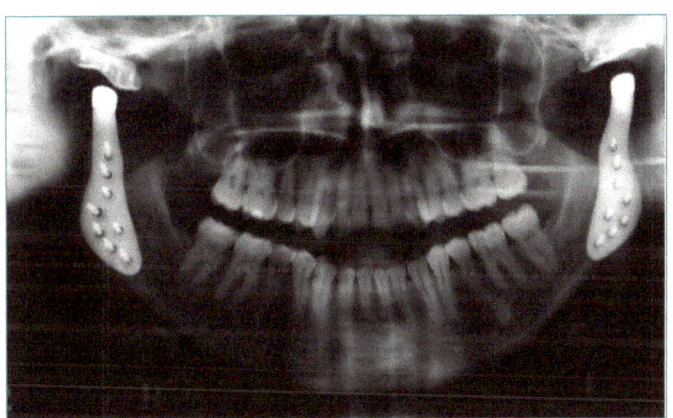

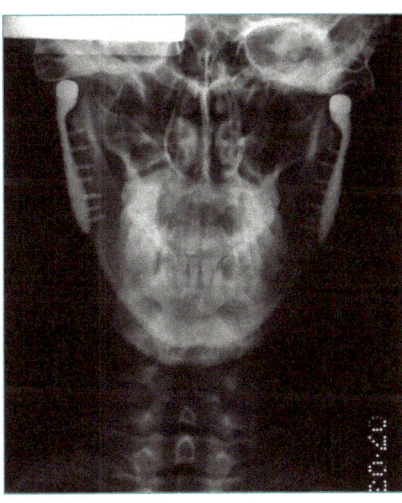

Figures 3.25 & 3.26: Postoperative OPG and PA mandible showing new bilateral temporomandibular joints. Note the condylar prosthesis is fixed to the ascending ramus of the mandible. Pictures courtesy of Mr. Andrew Sidebottom

3.4.4 TMJ DISLOCATION

Patients who present with a sudden-onset inability to close their jaw with their mouth in a wide-open position will most likely be suffering with a dislocated TMJ. Here, the condylar head has slipped forward over the articular eminence. There may be a prior history of TMJD or excessive mouth opening such as yawning or undergoing prolonged dental treatment. Patients are often distressed and may report previous similar episodes.

The earlier the jaw is relocated, generally the easier the procedure is to carry out. As soon as feasibly possible, one should attempt to relocate the jaw by applying sustained bilateral thumb pressure inside the mouth on the retromolar pads in order to manipulate the condyle under, and posterior to, the articular eminence of the temporal bone. The fingers are placed around the outside of the jaw to help stabilise it. If the TMJ is not relocated in a timely manner, or if there are too many unsuccessful attempts, this procedure becomes more challenging due to spasm and tightening of the masticatory muscles, and can often require intravenous sedation or even a GA with muscle relaxant to achieve joint reduction without causing excessive pain and stress to the patient.

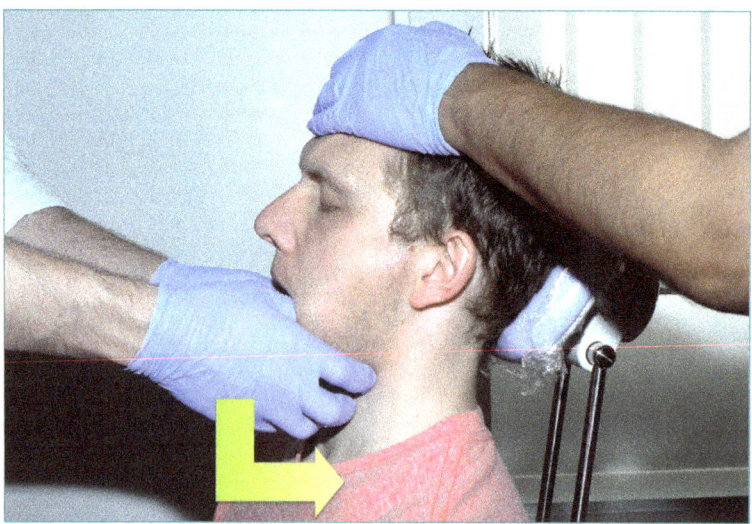

Figure 3.27: Reducing a dislocated mandible. Note support of patient's head and position of hands around mandible. Pressure is applied downwards to disengage the condyle from the eminence.

3.4.5 MECHANICAL OBSTRUCTION OF THE TMJ

Occasionally patients can present with insidious onset of evolving trismus and this can be because of hyperplasia of the coronoid process. (See Figure 3.28, 'coronoid hyperplasia' – look at the tip of the coronoid relative to the condylar head.) For those of you who are fascinated with rare presentations, this can be a manifestation of Jacob's disease – although not in this case! Jacob's disease is where a pseudo-joint is thought to form between the coronoid process and body of the zygoma.

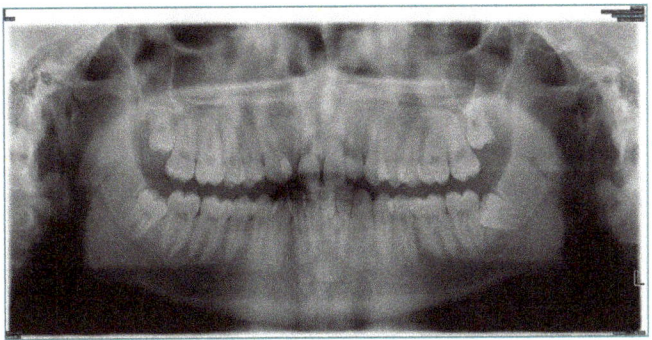

Figure 3.28: Photo of coronoid hyperplasia as seen on OPG (coronoid marked out on left side). This patient presented with an inability to open his mouth because of impingement of the coronoid on the zygoma. Picture courtesy of Miss Nabeela Ahmed

Treatment modalities in these cases can include coronoid release or coronoidectomy (where the coronoids are excised) and this can be undertaken via an intra- or extra-oral approach. The case above was treated via an intra-oral approach and the coronoids were excised as seen below.

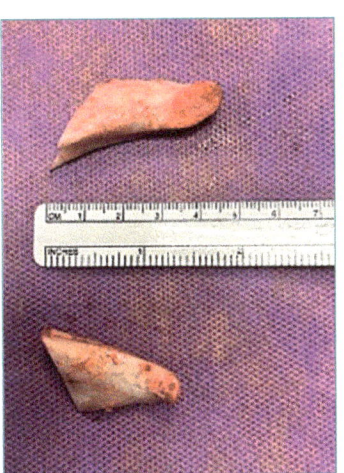

Figure 3.29: Photos of excised coronoid processes done via an intra-oral approach from previous case. On table, mouth opening improved immediately intra-operatively. Picture courtesy of Miss Nabeela Ahmed

Postoperatively, it is essential to achieve and maintain normal mouth opening; however, as the reader can appreciate, this is dependent on the timeframe over which the trismus has evolved. In difficult cases, a 'Therabite' appliance can be used by the patient at home to gradually increase their mouth opening in increments over time.

Like many other joints, TMJ disease can also be managed with the replacement of the joint and is a commonly performed operation for which there is NICE guidance. These patients are managed by specialist surgeons and replacement of the joint is not undertaken lightly. Assessment for such patients includes a CT scan (upon which the custom-made prosthesis is designed), patch testing to ensure there is no reactivity to any of the prosthetic joint components and an anaesthetic review (as joint destruction may be associated with systemic disease such as rheumatoid or psoriatic arthritis or complete trismus because of ankylosis after either trauma or infection). See Figure 3.30 for how a joint replacement is planned.

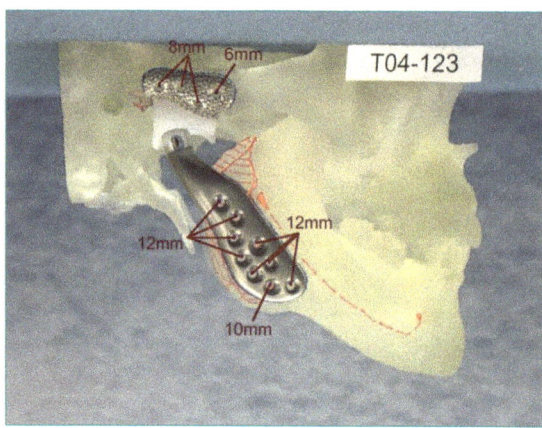

Figure 3.30: How a TMJ replacement is planned. This 3D model shows the level of the joint resection, path of the ID canal and length of screws required for fixation. Picture courtesy of Mr. Andrew Sidebottom

3.5 CYSTS OF THE JAW

The most common type of cyst you will encounter on a maxillofacial clinic will be a radicular cyst. However, a common reason for patients to be referred is the finding of an incidental cyst on OPG. They are considered as odontogenic or non-odontogenic in origin. Odontogenic cysts include radicular, dentigerous cysts and keratocystic odontogenic tumours. Other considerations when reviewing these should include the potential diagnosis of an ameloblastoma and potentially metastatic disease.

We'll briefly look at these, given the frequency with which they require management by the maxillofacial team.

3.5.1 RADICULAR CYSTS

These are often associated with non-vital teeth, and depending upon the size, may resolve spontaneously upon addressing the cause if less than 1cm in diameter – by either root filling or extracting the tooth. If this fails to address the situation, then often an apicectomy procedure is required, and enucleation and curettage of the associated cyst.

On occasion, extraction of the tooth fails to allow resolution of the cyst and this would be termed a residual cyst – and requires enucleation and curettage. This sectional OPG (Figure 3.31) demonstrates a residual cyst and the infill that has started to occur at four weeks.

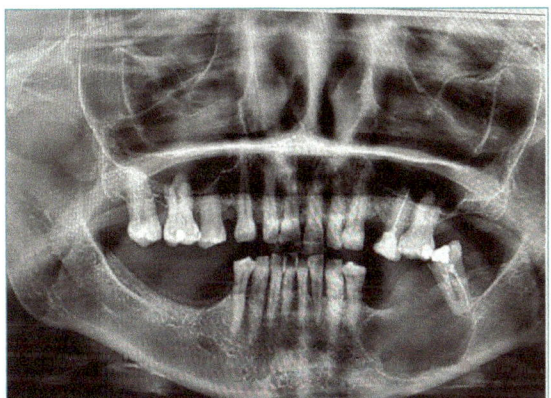

Figure 3.31a: Pre-op extraction and curettage of LL6 tooth and associated radicular cyst. Picture courtesy of Miss Nabeela Ahmed

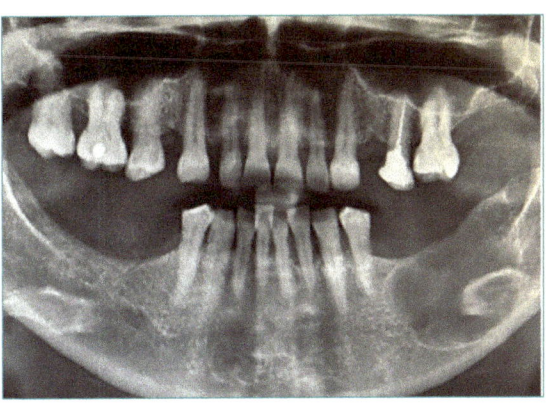

Figure 3.31b: Post-op extraction and curettage at six weeks. Note bony infill has started distal to the LL4 tooth. Picture courtesy of Miss Nabeela Ahmed

3.5.2 DENTIGEROUS CYSTS

These cysts, as you see in Figure 3.32, are always associated with the crown of an unerupted/impacted tooth (most commonly third molars) and treatment involves extraction of the tooth and curettage of the cyst. Once surgically treated they do not require follow-up (unless it's to monitor vitality of adjacent teeth, which the dentist can do).

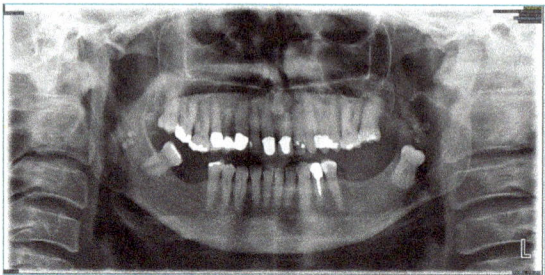

Figure 3.32a: Pre-op dentigerous cyst. Incidental tonsillitis both sides. Picture courtesy of Miss Claire Barrett

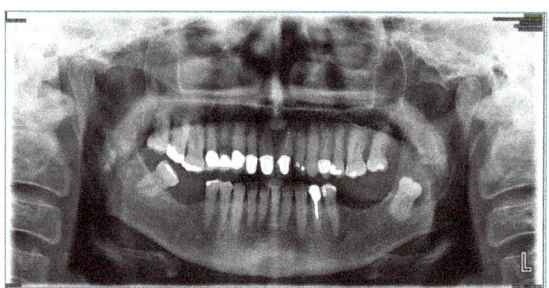

Figure 3.32b: Mid treatment for decompression. Notice how the cyst cavity has reduced. Picture courtesy of Miss Claire Barrett

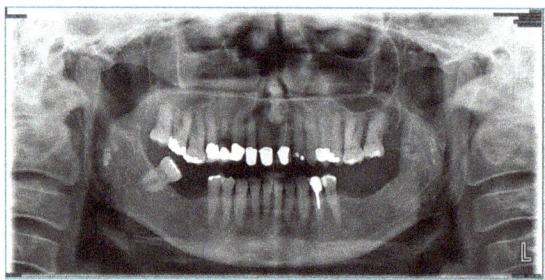

Figure 3.32c: Post treatment and formal enucleation and extraction of tooth. Picture courtesy of Miss Claire Barrett

3.5.3 ODONTOGENIC KERATOCYST

Odontogenic keratocysts were previously named keratocystic odontogenic tumours (KCOT) and the two terms are still used interchangeably. These are rare and benign but locally aggressive developmental cysts. Often found in the posterior mandible they can present and appear very similar to dentigerous cysts. They can appear in the maxilla, and when multiple cysts are present may be associated with Gorlin-Goltz syndrome.

There are a number of ways of treating these, ranging from decompression and enucleation, or enucleation with ostectomy and treatment of the residual cavity with Carnoy's solution or 5-Fluorouracil (5-FU). As they have a tendency to recur, they require follow-up long term. In a similar way to dentigerous cysts, they can be decompressed and then formally enucleated once smaller.

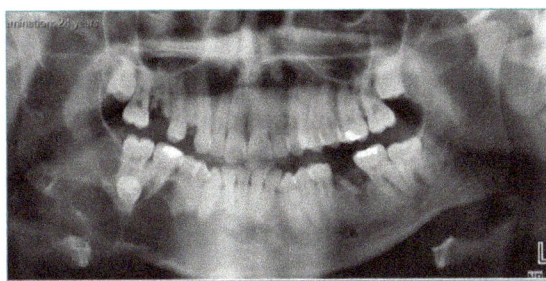

Figure 3.33a: A 24-year-old presenting with a right facial swelling. Note the 'soap bubble' multilocular lesion involving the right hemi-mandible. Picture courtesy of Mr. Rabin K.C. Singh

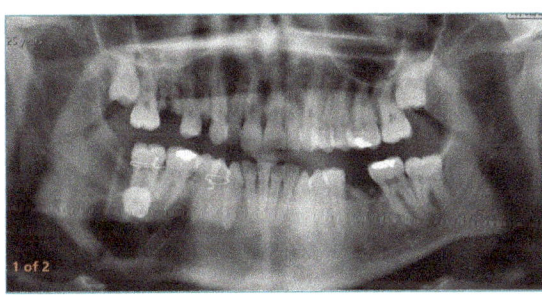

Figure 3.33b: Same patient, four months after two decompression tubes. You can see the endotracheal tube's shadow where it is wired into the cavity in the LR4 and LR7 region. There has been a significant change in the size of the lesion. Picture courtesy of Mr. Rabin K.C. Singh

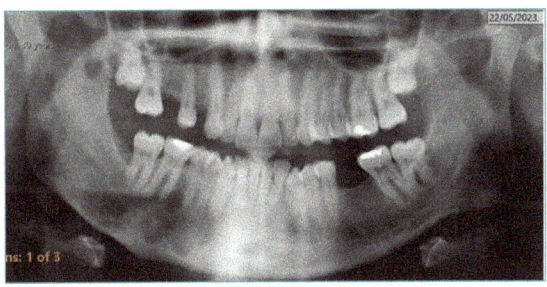

Figure 3.33c: Six years post enucleation of residual cyst and treatment with Carnoy's solution chemofixation. The radiolucent areas on the OPG show evidence of bone deposition on CT scan. This patient will remain under continual radiographic follow-up for 10 years. Picture courtesy of Mr. Rabin K.C. Singh

3.5.4 AMELOBLASTOMA

This is one of the commonest jaw tumours, which can be locally destructive. It can present as an asymptomatic unilocular or multilocular lesion of the jaw, with resorption and mobility of the teeth it is associated with. It should mandate an urgent referral to the maxillofacial unit when seen. Whilst these can present in a very similar way to KCOTs (as above) the main difference would be the resorption of any associated teeth and evidence clinically of buccal/lingual expansion. Whilst technically a benign tumour, if left untreated they have the potential for malignant transformation.

3.5.5 METASTATIC DISEASE

Bony metastases to the mandible can be a common occurrence for progressive/uncontrolled cancer of the breast, kidney, lung, thyroid, colon and prostate. It should be considered as cause for concern when patients present with new onset pain, which doesn't appear to be of dental origin, perhaps associated with paraesthesia. First-line imaging is often an OPG, and then CT, with a biopsy required to confirm the diagnosis.

Often, these present with a pathological fracture of the mandible, and can be challenging to manage alongside the need to evaluate and treat the cause. This is one of many reasons why a comprehensive and up-to-date medical history is required for patients that we see clinically, to ensure we consider all potential sequelae.

3.6 MEDICATION-RELATED OSTEONECROSIS OF THE JAWS (MRONJ)

MRONJ is characterised by non-healing exposed bone in a patient with a history of antiresorptive or antiangiogenic agents in the absence of radiation exposure to the head and neck region. You will almost certainly see this at some stage of your practising career.

The increasing use of bisphosphonates (such as alendronic/zolendronic acid) and other medications such as anti-TNF medications and RANK ligand inhibitors and antiangiogenics for a wide spectrum of disease from osteoporosis to bony metastases associated with cancer means that these patients require a holistic approach to management. There are guidelines in place for how these patients should be assessed and managed (www.sdcep.org.uk).

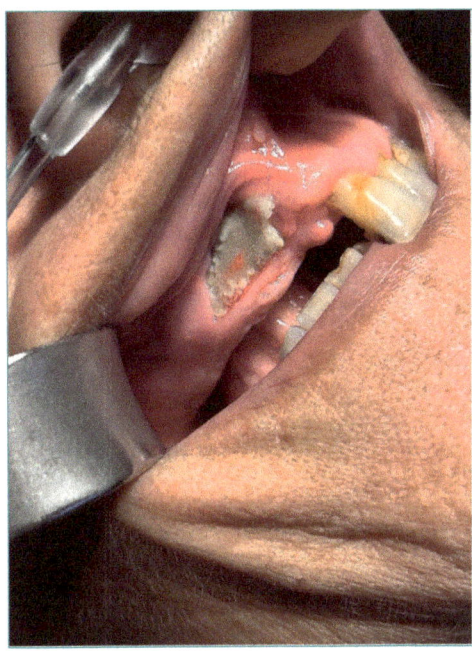

Figure 3.34: MRONJ of the UR3 region after extraction of tooth for a patient taking bisphosphonates for management of breast cancer metastatic disease. Note exposed necrotic bone extending beyond original extraction site with bleeding point centrally on curettage. Picture courtesy of Miss Nabeela Ahmed

The debate remains open as to whether stopping the causative medication (a so-called 'drug holiday') helps promote healing where there is exposed bone, and whether it would facilitate healing if a tooth did require extraction. Such patients are often referred into specialist services for management. Figure 3.34 demonstrates the catastrophic sequelae of the bone necrosis which can be triggered by the most innocuous of soft-tissue trauma. You need to be familiar with medications that can cause MRONJ and be mindful of undertaking any surgical procedure for patients taking them, and equally be suspicious if they present with unexplained dental pain/swelling.

3.7 OSTEORADIONECROSIS (ORN) OF THE JAWS

Osteoradionecrosis (ORN) is a serious side effect of radiation therapy for head and neck cancers. Any patient who has had treatment of oral/oropharyngeal cancer with either primary or adjunctive radiotherapy is at risk of developing osteoradionecrosis of the jaw. This is a direct result of the radiotherapy treatment and is a reason why all those having head and neck radiotherapy should have a dental screening before treatment.

Pre-radiotherapy assessment involves extraction of all teeth of poor prognosis which may be compromised by the effects of the radiotherapy (which affects the salivary glands and causes xerostomia – you'll recall one of the functions of saliva is lubrication and neutralisation of potential cariogenic insults).

Patients who have had radiotherapy may develop ORN in response to mild periodontal or periapical disease and the manifestations can be huge – resulting in necrosis of the jaw which may result in pain/discomfort and even pathological fracture. Teeth in this cohort of patients are often managed by the OMFS/OS team and should not be extracted in general dental practice.

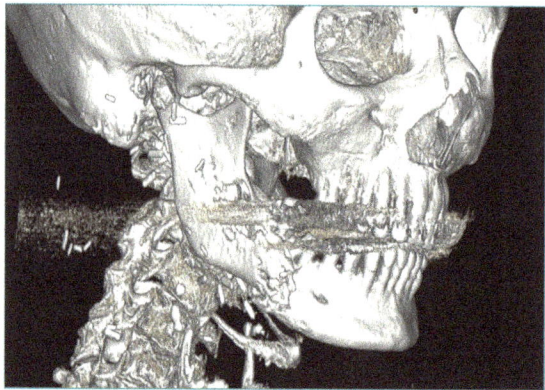

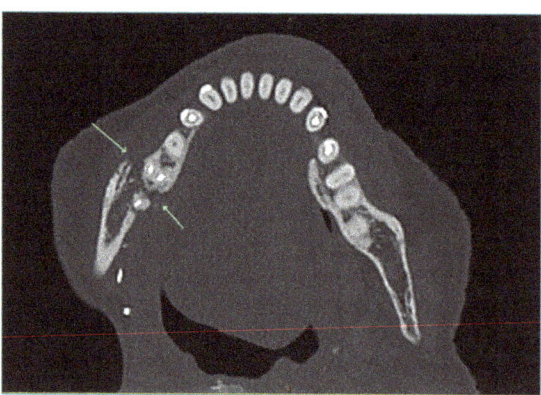

Figure 3.35: 3D reformat of a CT scan of a patient presenting with altered bite, pain and an orocutaneous fistula. The first image shows a right body fracture which can also be seen on the axial CT view (arrowed). Pictures courtesy of Mr. Muammar Abu-Serriah

This chapter has covered an extensive amount of material that will feature in your everyday practice as dentists. Please consider further reading and asking questions when you attend your OMFS and oral surgery placements.

CHAPTER 4: SALIVARY GLANDS, THE FACIAL NERVE AND FACIAL PAIN

4.1 ANATOMY

Saliva represents the start of the digestive process and mechanical lubrication of food within the mouth. In addition, it is protective to the oral mucosa and teeth. Aside from minor oral salivary glands, three paired major salivary glands produce the majority of saliva – the parotid, submandibular and sublingual glands.

Parotid glands – These glands predominantly produce a serous type of saliva. They are located on either side of the face, anterior to the ear, and extend downwards under the earlobe and around the posterior border of the mandible. Saliva produced by the parotid drains into the parotid (or 'Stenson's') duct, which pierces the buccinator muscle and opens into the oral cavity opposite the upper second molar tooth. When you look inside the mouth, you will see a small papilla at this site, which represents the duct opening.

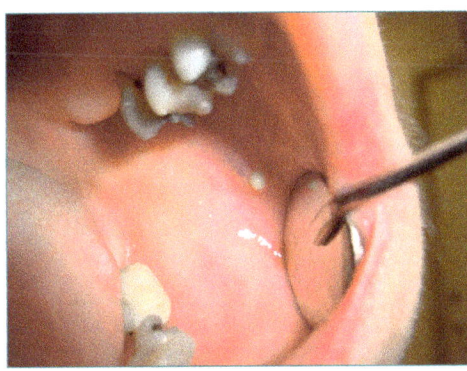

Figure 4.1: Here you can see the opening of the parotid duct opposite the upper second molar. Interestingly, frank pus is coming from the duct. This is usually in keeping with parotitis. Picture courtesy of Mr. Stephen Walsh

In terms of surgery, the most important anatomical characteristic of the parotid gland is its intimate relationship with the facial nerve, the branches of which run through it – dividing the gland into anatomically relevant superficial and deep lobes. Therefore, any surgical procedure involving the parotid gland (for example, a superficial parotidectomy) includes the risk of injury to the facial nerve. As the facial nerve supplies the muscles of facial expression, damage to it can clearly cause significant patient morbidity.

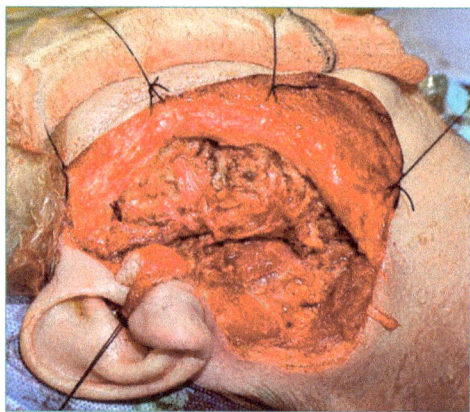

Figure 4.2: Here a tumour in the superficial lobe has been dissected carefully off the underlying facial nerve, which can be seen spreading out as branches from a main trunk. Underneath the nerve itself is the deep lobe of the parotid. Picture courtesy of Mr. Madan Ethunandan

Submandibular glands – These are located high up in the neck towards the angle of the mandible and wrap around the free edge of one of the muscles that forms the floor of the mouth – the mylohyoid. They produce a more mucous-like, thicker saliva, which drains into the oral cavity via the submandibular (or 'Wharton's') duct, which opens on either side of the lingual frenum. Examination of this gland requires bimanual palpation.

Sublingual glands – The last set of major salivary glands are the sublingual glands, which exist in the floor of the mouth. They are each the size of a walnut and drain either directly into the mouth or into the submandibular duct. Surgeons become concerned with the sublingual glands because the lingual nerve – supplying sensation and taste to the anterior two-thirds of the tongue – runs close by. Thus, any surgery to this gland carries a risk of damage to this nerve.

4.2 SALIVARY-GLAND PATHOLOGY

So what can go wrong with salivary glands? Like any glandular tissue, the salivary glands can be the site of a mass or tumour, grow in an abnormal fashion (become hypertrophic) or become obstructed (i.e. by a salivary stone).

4.2.1 SALIVARY TUMOURS

Salivary-gland tumours can be either benign or malignant. In general, there is an intriguing relationship between the size of a gland and the risk of a tumour within it being malignant – **the smaller the gland, the greater the chance of a malignant tumour**. To illustrate this point, approximately 20% of all parotid-gland lumps will be malignant, compared with 50% in the submandibular gland and 85% of sublingual-gland tumours. In other words, only 15% of sublingual-gland tumours are benign. That said, it is important to emphasise that salivary-gland cancers are rare, representing only 1% of malignant tumours of the head and neck. The 'rule of 80s' is a useful tool for any medical or dental student: 80% of salivary tumours are in the parotid, 80% of parotid tumours are benign and 80% of these are pleomorphic adenomas.

Most salivary tumours present as a painless mass – they are often slow growing, but some, particularly malignant tumours, can be painful or grow quite rapidly. It is important when assessing a lump that might originate in the salivary glands to note any presence of facial-nerve involvement or any cervical lymphadenopathy, as these are worrying signs of a more sinister pathology. As with any neck examination, this is completed by looking inside the mouth for any deep-lobe parotid-gland tumour extension which might be seen as a swelling in the lateral pharyngeal wall.

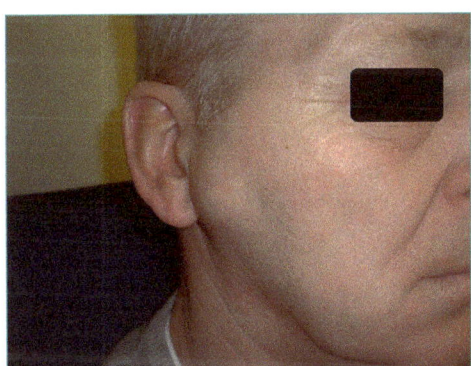

Figure 4.3: This patient presented with a slow-growing, painless mass in the right parotid. It is essential to assess the facial nerve in such patients! Picture courtesy of Mr. Stephen Walsh

A salivary-gland mass will routinely be assessed by an ultrasound scan (USS) with or without fine-needle aspiration cytology (FNAC), which is used to assess the cells aspirated from the mass under a microscope. Depending on the pathology, CT and MRI scans will also be used to give a more detailed view of the mass and its extension within the salivary gland. With malignant disease, USS, CT and MRI can all be helpful in determining any lymph-node involvement. As with all head and neck cancers, malignant salivary-gland cancers are staged using the TNM system, where the size of the tumour (T), the presence of cervical lymph nodes (N) and the development of distant metastasis (M) are all important factors that determine management and prognosis. This information often dictates whether these tumours can be removed surgically or require other adjunctive treatment, such as removal of the draining lymph nodes in the neck or chemo-radiotherapy.

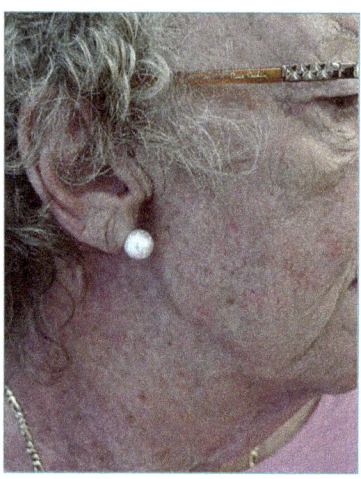

Figure 4.4: This patient presented with a palpable lump in the right parotid gland. Picture courtesy of Mr. Madan Ethunandan

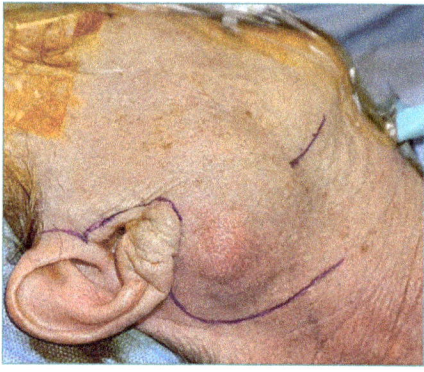

Figure 4.5: An incision is made around the ear, into the neck. We do our best to hide the incisions in such a way as to make them inconspicuous. Picture courtesy of Mr. Madan Ethunandan

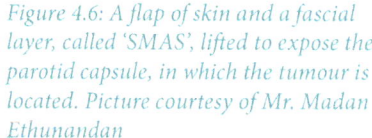

Figure 4.6: A flap of skin and a fascial layer, called 'SMAS', lifted to expose the parotid capsule, in which the tumour is located. Picture courtesy of Mr. Madan Ethunandan

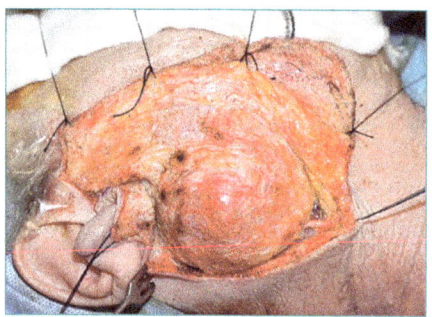

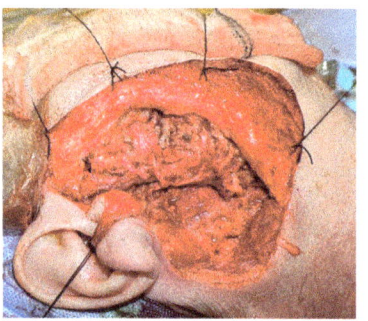

Figure 4.7: The tumour is dissected carefully off the underlying facial nerve, which can be seen spreading out as branches from a main trunk. Picture courtesy of Mr. Madan Ethunandan

A mass in the submandibular or sublingual salivary glands (either benign or malignant) will be surgically removed via excision of the gland itself – a relatively common procedure. However, when you get to the parotid gland, things start to get more interesting and controversial. The jury is still out as to the best treatment plan for a benign superficial-lobe parotid mass (i.e. a pleomorphic adenoma), with evidence for and against removing only the lump itself (termed an 'extra-capsular dissection', a less-invasive procedure) or removing the entirety of the superficial lobe (aka a 'superficial parotidectomy'). The latter procedure involves formal identification of the main trunks of the facial nerve in the first instance, thus in theory minimising the risk of facial-nerve injury. Surgery to a malignant parotid mass will require a clear margin of tissue to be excised in addition to the mass itself, and in some cases may require sacrifice of the facial nerve.

The advantages of extra-capsular dissection are that it can be undertaken via a smaller incision and that it reduces the risk of gustatory sweating (Frey's syndrome), which can occur after parotid surgery.

4.2.2 OBSTRUCTIVE SALIVARY-GLAND DISEASE

The salivary ducts are prone to becoming blocked by stones that can precipitate from the saliva within them (sialolithiasis). Their formation is multifactorial, but when they grow large enough, they can occlude the duct system within the gland. This is classically described as 'mealtime syndrome'. Here, when patients salivate – typically when they are about to eat – and the saliva production increases, the saliva flow is impeded by their stone, causing a build-up of back-pressure with the gland, resulting in pain. Often, patients report a foul discharge or even a gritty sensation in their mouth. This pattern is repeated whenever the patient eats. Sometimes, because saliva is stagnant in the blocked gland, the gland can become inflamed or infected, which can require urgent management, requiring antibiotics or even surgical drainage. Narrowing or 'stenosis' of salivary ducts can also present with obstructive symptoms.

An ultrasound scan (USS) is a useful first-line investigation for patients with these problems, but other radiographic techniques can also be used. For example, a sialogram is an investigation whereby radiopaque contrast material is introduced through the duct orifice with a blunt-ended catheter to delineate the duct anatomy and more clearly mark out any obstruction (or stenosis). Some surgeons use endoscopic techniques to identify and retrieve stones from the duct or can consider direct intra-oral stone release. In the case of the submandibular and sublingual glands, when stones are large or located further towards the gland and difficult to access, we usually have no option but to surgically remove the entire gland. Endoscopic guided stone retrieval is an increasingly popular way of addressing this problem and resultant gland preservation.

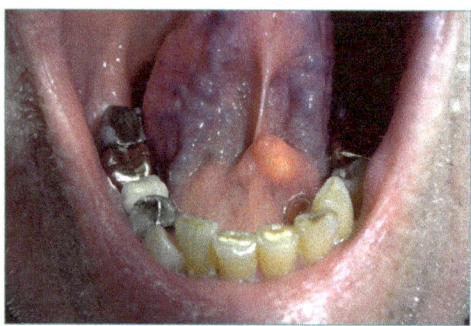

Figure 4.8: Here you can see a salivary stone or calculus in the floor of a mouth, just beneath the surface of the mucosa. They travel along the path of the submandibular duct but sometimes get trapped. Picture courtesy of Mr. Stephen Walsh

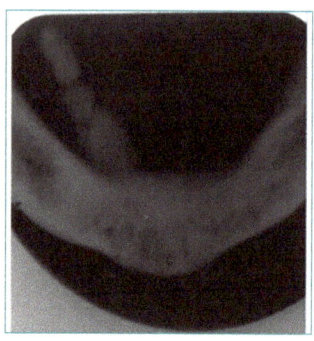

Figure 4.9: Sometimes salivary calculi or stones are visible on plain film x-rays. This is called an 'occlusal radiograph' and clearly shows a stone in the floor of the mouth. Picture courtesy of Mr. Andrew Sidebottom

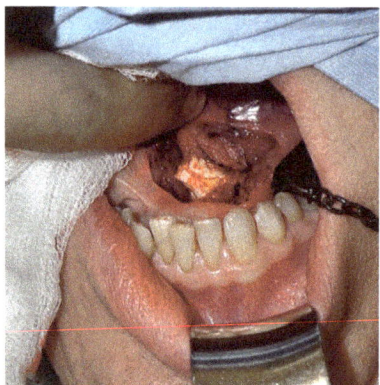

Figure 4.10: This is a different patient, who would have presented with a blocked right submandibular duct. Incising into the floor of the mouth allows retrieval of the stone. Picture courtesy of Mr. Madan Ethunandan

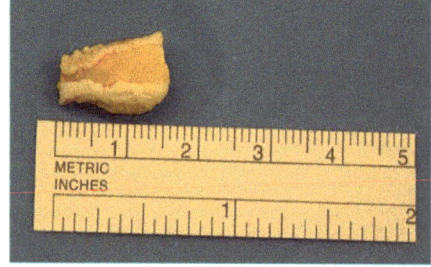

Figure 4.11: This is the same calculus. Very much like renal calculi, these can cause obstructive symptoms and cause extensive swelling in the associated gland. Picture courtesy of Mr. Madan Ethunandan

4.2.3 SALIVARY GLAND TRAUMA

As with any of the facial structures, salivary glands can be involved in a traumatic injury, either directly (e.g. from a stab wound) or indirectly, via blunt-force trauma. As discussed elsewhere, a mucocele – one of the most common small lumps occurring in the mouth – is a result of trauma to a minor salivary gland, often on the lip. Sometimes, when this affects the sublingual gland, it leads to a dramatic-looking, bluish swelling in the floor of the mouth, which resembles a frog's neck and has been accordingly termed a ranula.

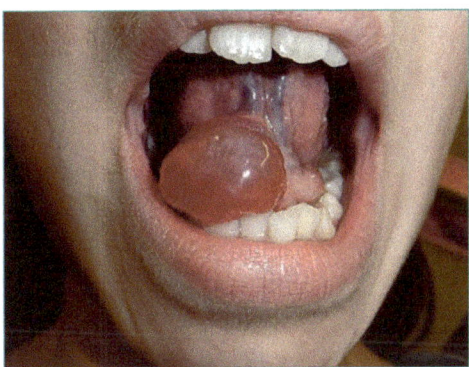

Figure 4.12: This is a ranula, a collection of saliva in the floor of the mouth. Sometimes they can herniate into the neck, which is known as a plunging ranula. Picture courtesy of Mr. Madan Ethunandan

Saliva can leak out directly from the gland into the neighbouring tissues, creating a salivary collection or sialocele. Often this is a result of iatrogenic trauma (i.e. previous surgery causing damage to the gland), which commonly affects the parotid gland. Another common complication that might arise from parotid surgery or injury is Frey's syndrome, sometimes described as 'gustatory sweating'. Normally, the parotid gland is supplied by parasympathetic secretomotor fibres from the glossopharyngeal nerve (via the otic ganglion). The skin's sweat glands are supplied by sympathetic nerve fibres (from the thoracic ganglion). Injury/surgery to the parotid gland and overlying skin means that there is 'cross wiring' of salivary secretomotor fibres with secretomotor fibres of sweat glands, such that upon eating, the patient suffers from excessive sweating.

4.3 FACIAL PAIN

A patient presenting with facial pain or altered sensation can be extremely difficult to diagnose and treat. While organic causes may be obvious and can be treated accordingly, there may be a strong psychological component that can be difficult to address. However, dental pathology is still the most common cause of facial pain and a detailed history and examination warrants prompt assessment by the patient's dentist.

If the pain is not characteristic of a dental cause, then a thorough pain history is required. With an understanding of the different aetiologies of facial pain, your history will become more focused. Is the pain intermittent or episodic in nature? Does it 'shoot' down the face in the distribution of the trigeminal nerve? Is the pain there at night? Does it wake the patient from sleep? Is the pain associated with earache or sinusitis? In addition, a past medical history should include asking about other neurological disorders and mental health. Examination should include the face, mouth, nasal cavity, neck and cranial nerves.

Non-dental Benign Facial Pain Syndromes

Unfortunately, this list is extensive and, to confuse matters further, specialists in this area have a habit of changing the terminology for such conditions every few years. Below, we discuss some of the common causes of facial pain, which are frequently referred to OMFS units across the country.

4.3.1 TEMPOROMANDIBULAR DISORDER

Temporomandibular joint disorder (TMJD), as covered in section 3.4, is an umbrella term describing dysfunction of the temporomandibular joint and associated muscular apparatus that causes pain and symptoms of the jaw joint and face. It is important to diagnose this correctly as the vast majority of cases can be managed non-operatively with minimal intervention aside from the provision of a dental splint/bite raising appliance.

4.3.2 TRIGEMINAL NEURALGIA

Trigeminal neuralgia is an extremely painful condition caused by irritation to the trigeminal nerve. Classically, it produces a sharp 'lightning' (or 'shooting') pain in the distribution of one of the divisions of the trigeminal nerve (ophthalmic, maxillary, mandibular) and typically occurs in 'sporadic bursts' lasting seconds to hours at a time. The pain often has a specific trigger (e.g. physical touch to a trigger area or a change in temperature) and does not cross the midline. Despite being brief in nature, it can be debilitating and is often described as the worst pain the patient has ever experienced. Patients live in fear of it reoccurring and certainly should be screened like all chronic pain conditions regarding the impact on their mood and suicidal ideation.

Examination is fairly unremarkable; however, patients with triggers may become increasingly anxious that you may provoke an episode of pain by examining them. Obviously, all dental causes of pain need to be excluded first.

As part of the diagnostic arsenal, cross-sectional imaging, most notably MRI, is invaluable to exclude space-occupying lesions (SOL) or blood vessels compressing the trigeminal nerve in the cerebellopontine angle or, in the case of patients under the age of 40 years, for the assessment for evidence of multiple sclerosis.

Trigeminal neuralgia can be managed either medically with carbamazepine, or surgically, often dependent on the underlying cause. In medically refractory cases, if the pain can be isolated to a single division of the trigeminal nerve, then targeted treatments such as direct cryotherapy or microvascular decompression of the nerve root have been shown to be beneficial. Furthermore, in the acute setting, the use of a mixture of short- and long-acting local anaesthetics can be both diagnostic and (temporarily) therapeutic to the patient.

4.3.3 ATYPICAL FACIAL PAIN AND BURNING MOUTH SYNDROME

In contrast to trigeminal neuralgia, atypical facial pain and burning mouth syndrome (oral dysaesthesia) represent facial pain syndromes with no organic cause, and a strong psychological component. The pain and symptoms of atypical facial pain follow no myofascial or nerve distribution, are varying in character and with no recognisable pattern, but crucially, they do not disturb eating or sleep. It more commonly affects females, particularly those who are middle aged, and there can be an association with hormonal changes associated with the menopause. As a diagnosis of exclusion, a detailed history, followed by an unremarkable clinical examination, can aid diagnosis.

Patients with burning mouth syndrome may also present with altered or a metallic taste. On examination, the soft tissue of the mouth will appear normal. Diagnosis is by exclusion – including blood tests for haematological and nutritional deficiencies including FBC, B12, folate and ferritin, and diabetes mellitus and excluding candida infection, all of which can cause a burning sensation of the mouth.

Any of the above should be treated before a formal diagnosis of burning mouth syndrome is made. Patients with atypical facial pain or burning mouth syndrome are typically treated after exclusion of pathology on examination, with reassurance, symptomatic relief (i.e. using analgesic mouthwash) and on occasions low-dose tricyclic antidepressants may be warranted.

4.3.4 POST-HERPETIC NEURALGIA

Shingles, or herpes zoster, is caused by reactivation of the varicella-zoster virus. On the rest of the body its distribution follows the dermatomes, resulting in an eruption of an isolated and localised vesicular rash. On the face, it tends to be distributed along one of the three divisions of the trigeminal nerve, with no crossing of the midline.

As the virus can reside within neural tissue, it can cause damage with subsequent intermittent neuralgic pain along the distribution of that nerve. Patients can also show some degree of scarring in the affected disease areas. Managing this can be incredibly challenging. A number of drugs are used, including gabapentin, tricyclic antidepressants (such as amitriptyline) and anticonvulsants (like carbamazepine); however, in most cases the pain is refractory.

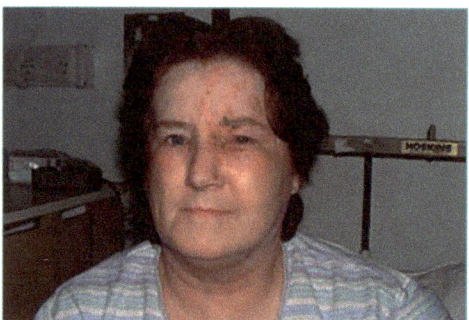

Figure 4.13: This patient presented with herpes zoster in the left ophthalmic division of the trigeminal nerve (V1). Note that this does not cross the midline. This patient should also be assessed by our ophthalmology colleagues to assess the globe itself. Picture courtesy of Mr. Andrew Sidebottom

4.4 FACIAL PALSY

The term 'facial palsy' means weakness or total paralysis of the muscles of facial expression and can be due to many different causes. The commonest is Bell's palsy, which is usually idiopathic (but can be inflammatory or post-viral) with a short onset (days).

Ramsay Hunt syndrome occurs when a post-herpetic neuropathy presents with facial weakness and vesicles in the external ear canal. Other rarer causes to be aware of include congenital problems, other neurological disease (such as Guillain-Barré and multiple sclerosis), tumours (e.g. a skull-base/brain tumour or nerve sheath tumour such as a schwannoma), trauma to the face/nerve, surgery itself (e.g. parotid or TMJ surgery), metabolic disorders (such as hyperthyroidism and diabetes mellitus) and autoimmune conditions.

Facial palsy is graded by using the House–Brackmann scale, which ranges from 1 (normal facial function in all areas) to 6 (total paralysis). When it

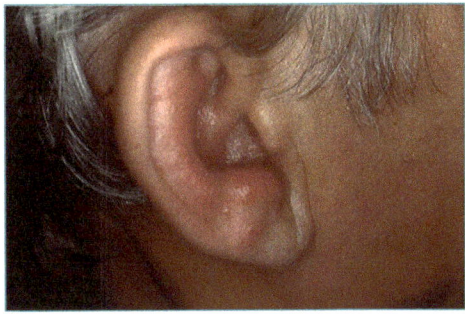

Figure 4.14: This patient presented with right-sided facial palsy. Examination of the right ear identified vesicles in the external auditory meatus. The diagnosis: Ramsay Hunt syndrome. Picture courtesy of Mr. Andrew Sidebottom

occurs, the most immediate concern is to protect the affected eye from drying out by placing a protective eye shield or taping the eye shut. If untreated, this can lead to corneal abrasion/ulceration (due to loss of eye closure). Depending on the underlying cause, systemic steroids and antivirals may be considered, although the evidence base is equivocal.

Surgery is required urgently if the nerve is likely to have been traumatically severed (e.g. by a facial laceration or stabbing injury). This would involve repair of the severed nerve ends under a microscope with incredibly fine sutures. Any penetrating laceration to the face in the area overlying the parotid gland mandates assessment of the facial nerve.

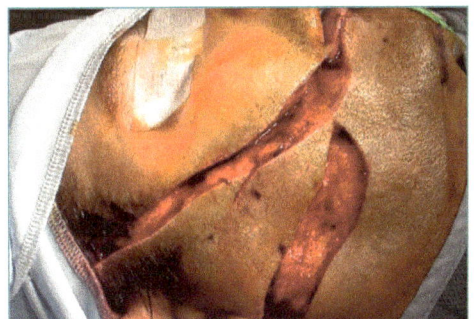

Figure 4.15: This patient suffered significant facial injuries as a result of interpersonal violence. The patient presented with facial paralysis, suggesting the facial-nerve branches had been severed. Picture courtesy of Professor P. Brennan

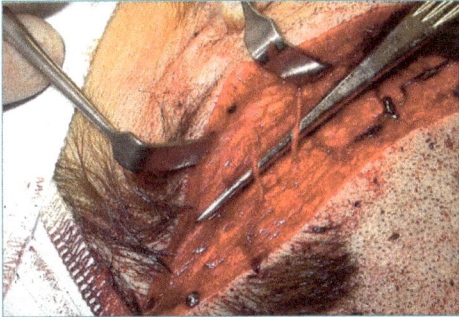

Figure 4.16: The wound was explored urgently. Here you can see two branches of the facial nerve which were repaired with the use of incredibly fine sutures under a powerful microscope. Picture courtesy of Professor P. Brennan

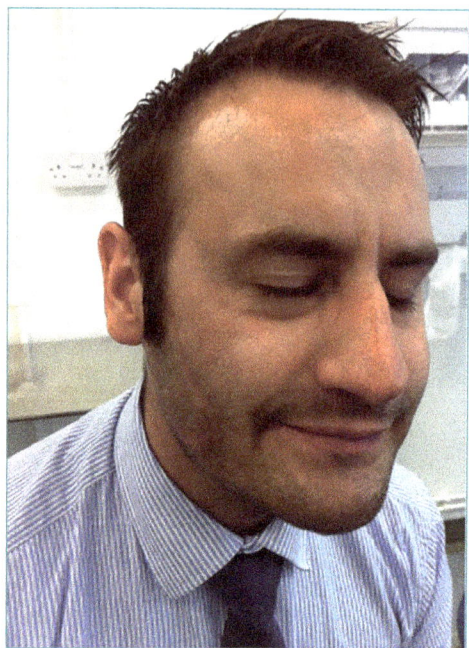

Figure 4.17: This is the same patient nine months post-injury. Notice both the symmetry in his smile, but also his ability to close his eye. This is an essential role of the facial nerve. Picture courtesy of Professor P. Brennan

In cases of persistent nerve palsy or in those who present late, 'facial reanimation' may be required. This may involve 'static procedures' (such as forehead, brow and/or face lifts). Alternatively, 'dynamic' procedures may be performed, which include functional muscle transfer of masticatory (chewing) muscles to help with facial movement, functional masticatory (masseter) nerve transfer to facial muscles, use of nerve grafts to repair/re-innervate the affected facial nerve, or even the transfer of free muscle flaps. Such flaps include auto-transplantation of the gracilis muscle from the groin to the face, with anastomosis (microsurgical connection) of the artery, vein and nerve supply to the corresponding blood vessels and viable motor nerve in the face/neck.

These unique dynamic reanimation surgeries have evolved over the last couple of decades with advances in microsurgery and are increasingly becoming the gold-standard treatment for severe persistent facial palsy.

CHAPTER 5: SOFT TISSUES AND THE NECK

5.1 FACIAL LACERATIONS AND NECK WOUNDS

Soft-tissue Wounds

The head and neck, and particularly the face, are a frequent and exposed site for soft-tissue injury. Common causes include interpersonal violence, sporting injuries, mechanical falls, animal bites and road-traffic collisions. In OMFS, we see a LOT of facial lacerations and incised wounds. On a daily basis, an OMFS trainee/junior surgeon will be in the emergency department (ED) suturing facial lacerations and treating patients with facial soft-tissue injuries. Technically speaking, a 'laceration' is defined as a break in the skin caused by a blunt-force or shearing trauma and an 'incised wound' is caused by a sharp object or implement, such as a knife. However, in day-to-day practice it has become commonplace to call the majority of injuries 'lacerations', regardless of the aetiology.

The take-home message from this chapter is that regardless of how minor the injury may appear, a thorough ATLS approach to assessment is mandatory. It is common, even in seemingly mild injuries, to have underlying injuries to deep vital or bony structures. The drama from an actively bleeding facial laceration may be masking a much more serious injury and a judicious assessment will avoid potential complications later on.

5.1.1 SIMPLE SOFT-TISSUE LACERATIONS/WOUNDS

In most instances, simple lacerations or wounds can be thoroughly washed, debrided and closed at the time of presentation and assessment – either under LA in the ED or sometimes requiring a GA in theatre. There are a number of factors that must be considered when deciding if a laceration is amenable to closure.

Even before you have examined the patient, the history of the mechanism of injury should guide your management. For example, if a patient reports being '*stabbed with a knife*', you should consider underlying structures and potential damage to neurovascular structures, as well as the need for tetanus and antibiotic prophylaxis. The size and shape of the knife, whilst interesting from a forensic aspect, does not factor into the urgency of assessment. These are all factors that will impact the injury and management. Also ask specifically about risk of wound contamination – for example, trauma on a muddy sports field or a bite from a wild/unvaccinated animal. Factors such as these may point you towards a course of prophylactic antibiotics or an even-more-thorough wound washout under a GA. ALWAYS check the tetanus status of the patient, and if in doubt or in higher-risk/soil-contaminated wounds, give a tetanus booster (the BNF provides full guidelines for this).

When taking your history, as with all facial trauma, it is important to fully assess the cause of injury, in order to rule out any worrying precipitating factors. Did the patient collapse? If so, why? Will they need a thorough cardiovascular assessment by the medical team? If the injuries appear consistent with physical assault, are there any safety/safeguarding issues to raise? Always consider the issue of domestic violence.

When you examine the wound, you may first need to clean it and the surrounding area to get a clearer view of the depth of penetration and surrounding soft-tissue injury or trauma to local structures.

5.1.2 DEEP SOFT-TISSUE INJURIES

When we talk about 'deep facial injuries' we are concerned about injuries to vital structures beneath the skin. Obviously, there are a lot of important anatomical structures within the face. Superficial blood vessels, such as the facial artery and vein, and superficial temporal vessels can cause significant bleeding. In deep facial lacerations/wounds, broadly speaking we are immediately concerned about the facial nerve and parotid duct. This is because these are structures that may need complex microsurgical reconstruction and the wound should be temporarily cleaned and packed first, and closed at a secondary procedure (as we saw in the previous chapter – see Figure 4.15).

The location of the parotid duct can be identified using facial surface landmarks. If you draw an imaginary line from the tragus of the ear to mid-upper lip, the parotid duct lies in the middle third of this line (as seen in red in Figure 5.1). Deep wounds in this region need examination inside the mouth to check that saliva is still discharging from the parotid-duct orifice – which, as mentioned previously, is found adjacent to the second maxillary molar.

The facial nerve should be examined *before* injecting local anaesthetic. All five divisions (temporal, zygomatic, buccal, marginal mandibular and cervical) should be examined and their function clearly documented in the patient's notes. Recall your anatomy: the cervical branch supplies the platysma muscle in the neck. As a rule of thumb, any potential facial-nerve injury in front of a vertical line drawn through the lateral canthus of the eye is considered

AN ILLUSTRATED GUIDE

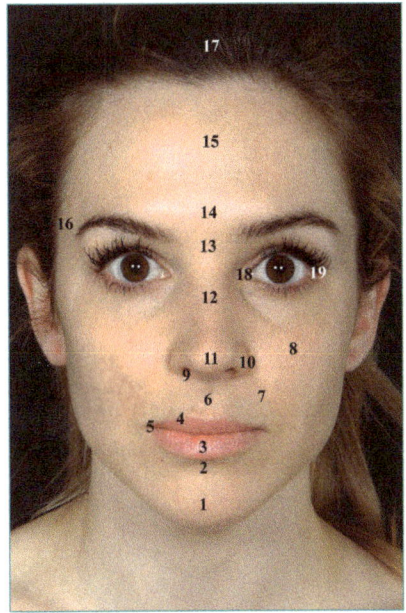
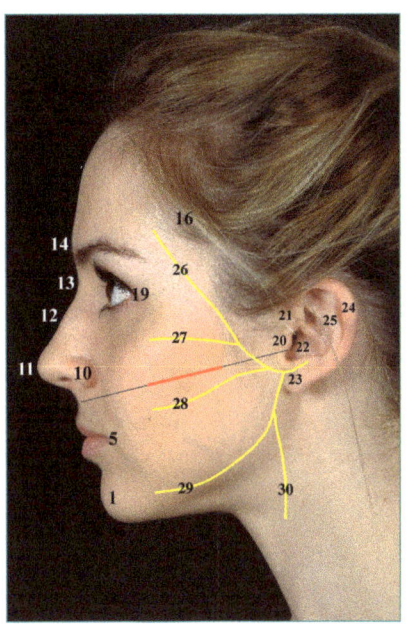

Figure 5.1: (a) Anterior view of surface anatomy of face. (b) Lateral view of surface anatomy of face, with representation of facial nerve (yellow line) and parotid duct (red line – middle third of line drawn from inferior tragus to mid-point of philtrum).

1. Chin
2. Labio-mental groove
3. Vermillion of lower lip
4. Vermillion border of upper lip
5. Oral commissure
6. Philtrum
7. Naso-labial groove
8. Cheek
9. Nares (nostril)
10. Ala of nose
11. Nasal tip
12. Dorsum/bridge of nose
13. Nasion
14. Glabella
15. Forehead
16. Temple
17. Scalp
18. Medial canthus
19. Lateral canthus
20. Tragus
21. External auditory meatus
22. Conchal bowl
23. Lobe
24. Helix
25. Antihelix
26. Temporal branch of facial nerve
27. Zygomatic branch of facial nerve
28. Buccal branch of facial nerve
29. Marginal mandibular branch of facial nerve
30. Cervical branch of facial nerve

low risk – the reason being that in this region the nerve has divided into smaller branches, so injury is potentially less serious. Any repair of such a small branch would be very difficult, if not impossible, even for the best microvascular surgeon around. A deep laceration posterior to this safe zone has a higher risk of cutting a named branch or even the trunk of the facial nerve and should therefore be examined more thoroughly. If in doubt, you should always have a low threshold for contacting a senior.

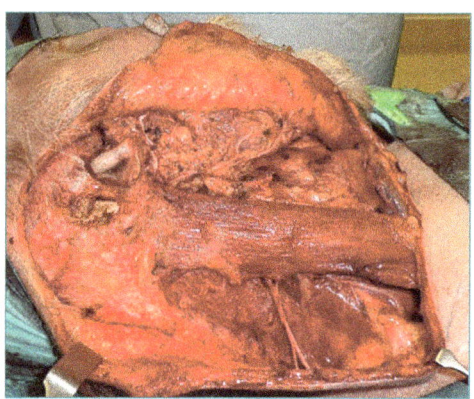

Figure 5.2: This is not a trauma patient, but the picture shows the path of the facial nerve and also the accessory nerve. In cancer and trauma patients, OMF surgeons spend time finding and protecting these. Picture courtesy of Mr. Madan Ethunandan

Penetrating Neck Injuries

In OMFS, we also accept referrals for penetrating neck injuries. Even with a lay appreciation of anatomy, it's clear to see that any penetrating injury to the neck (i.e. deep to the platysma muscle) has significant potential for injury to major neurovascular structures. Unlike lymph-node levels, the neck is divided into trauma zones I–III, with different vital structures at increased risk in each zone. This classification system is described by Monson, and can help triage the severity of the injury and guide assessment and resuscitation. The zones are:

- Zone I – From clavicles to cricoid cartilage
- Zone II – From cricoid cartilage to angle of mandible
- Zone III – From angle of mandible to base of skull.

If you are a junior trainee assessing a potential penetrating neck injury, you should call for help immediately. While a slight oversimplification, any patient with 'hard signs' (unstable observations and active haemorrhage) of a vascular injury should go to theatre straight away, whereas clinical suspicion alone may warrant a CT angiogram first to assess potential vascular injury. Injury to the common carotid or internal carotid artery (which is less likely because, as the name suggests, this is deep to the external carotid) requires input from

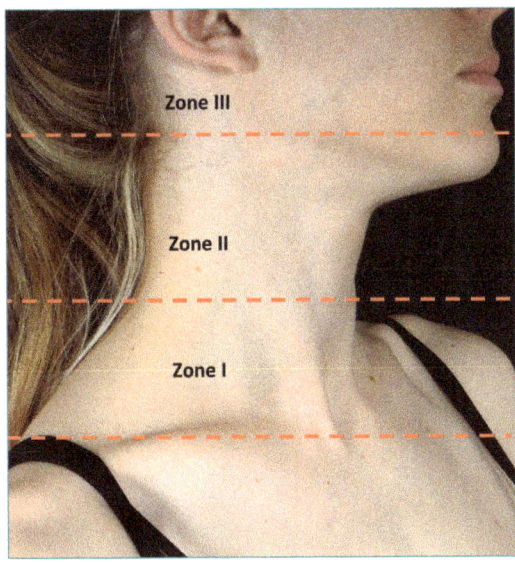

Figure 5.3: Lateral view of neck with markings for zones I–III

vascular surgeons. Given the increase in penetrating injuries of the neck, there are well-defined criteria on how these patients are managed and which teams are invited to attend the initial presentation (for neck injuries, these will include OMFS and ENT where practical).

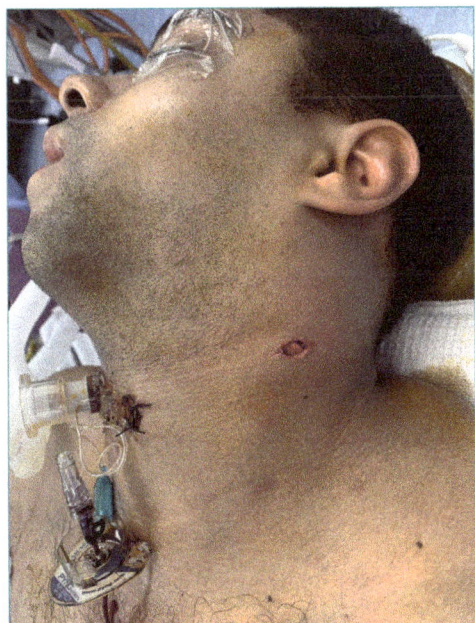

Figure 5.4: This patient presented with a stabbing to the neck. Whilst the wound only appears small, it is the damage to underlying structures and potential for bleeding in and around the neck that are of concern. Note that he has had a temporary tracheostomy placed to protect his airway. Pictures courtesy of Lieutenant Colonel Johno Breeze

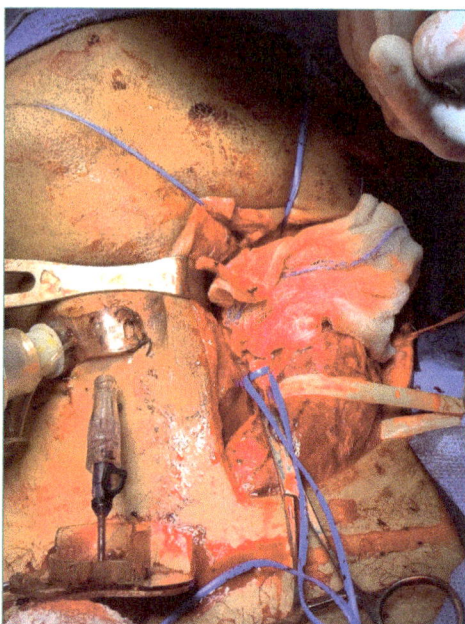

Figure 5.5: As well as securing this patient's airway with a temporary tracheostomy, OMF surgeons had to isolate the carotid artery to manage the underlying haemorrhage. Pictures courtesy of Lieutenant Colonel Johno Breeze

5.1.3 BITES

Bites from dogs, cats and, yes, even humans are grossly contaminated and carry a significant risk of infection. In addition, animals such as dogs are capable of significant forces, so crush injuries, tissue loss and underlying skeletal injury should always be considered. Cats on the other hand (with their sharp teeth) are more likely to cause puncture-type wounds, which on initial examination may appear innocuous, but in the depth of the wound there may be significant contamination.

The key to managing any form of bite is copious irrigation and debridement of the wound as required. Owing to the rich head and neck blood supply, if one is happy, primary closure of such wounds under a LA after a thorough washout is perfectly reasonable. However, a delayed approach can also sometimes be adopted, particularly if there is associated tissue loss – at this stage, local flaps and skin grafts will not be appropriate (given the potential risk of infection). All bites should be given prophylactic antibiotics, and local hospital guidelines are available in such instances.

5.2 NECK LUMPS

Most hospitals in the UK have a head and neck lump clinic, to which patients will be referred from primary care with a lump or mass requiring investigation. These clinics are often run jointly by OMFS and ENT. As a dental student, the concept of neck lumps can be daunting, especially when reading textbooks with long lists of possible causes. While you should be aware of all of these (especially for exams!), in clinical practice the common causes are much fewer. The majority of neck lumps seen in clinic will be related to lymph-node pathology, with the major concern being metastasis from undiagnosed head and neck cancer.

Assessment in a specialised clinic will comprise history, thorough examination and (if services allow) an immediate ultrasound scan (USS) with or without fine-needle aspiration cytology (FNAC) for pathological assessment. The best approach to classifying the aetiology of a neck lump is to divide causes into inflammatory, congenital or neoplastic.

5.2.1 INFLAMMATORY INCLUDING TISSUE SPACE INFECTIONS

Cervical lymphadenopathy secondary to infection is a common presentation. The head and neck have a wealth of lymph nodes (they can contain as many as 300 of the 800 or so nodes found throughout the body), which become enlarged, tender and palpable during times of infection. Common causes are: tonsillitis/peri-tonsillar abscess (quinsy), dental infection, pharyngitis, mastoiditis, otitis externa and otitis media, as well as skin pathology including acne.

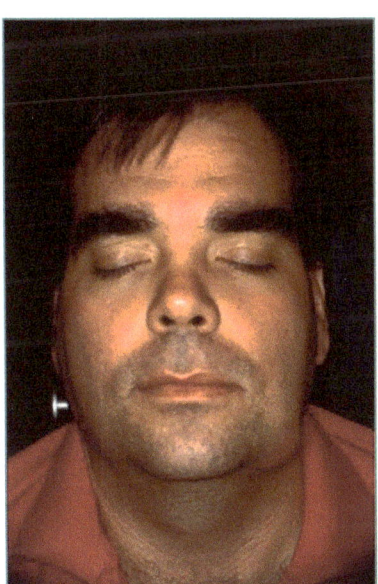

Figure 5.6: This patient presented with a chronic dental sinus secondary to dental abscess. The patient presented with lymphadenopathy, which resolved once the offending tooth was removed. Picture courtesy of Mr. Andrew Sidebottom

There are a number of 'fascial' layers within the head and neck that you should be aware of. Dental infections can cause extensive facial and neck swellings as the infection spreads unchallenged between these fascial spaces. There are a number of potential spaces that are in continuity with the mouth, and if infection spreads into these channels it can cause trismus, dysphagia and even potential threat to the airway. Ludwig's angina is a potentially fatal bilateral submandibular and sublingual cellulitis usually caused by a dental source. Patients often present with gross facial and neck swelling, difficulty swallowing their own saliva, a raised floor of mouth and looking systemically unwell – untreated, this can be rapidly fatal! Urgent intervention is required, usually in the form of a surgical airway and decompression of the submandibular and sublingual spaces, followed by a stay in the intensive care unit.

You should be familiar with the assessment of patients with facial swelling and consider that acute presentations, with rapid onset, associated trismus and systemic signs (such as increased heart rate and temperature), should prompt referral to the local OMFS unit for further evaluation and management. These remain life threatening, as the inability to open the mouth fully associated with any neck swelling may progress and cause airway compression which can be difficult to manage in the presence of trismus.

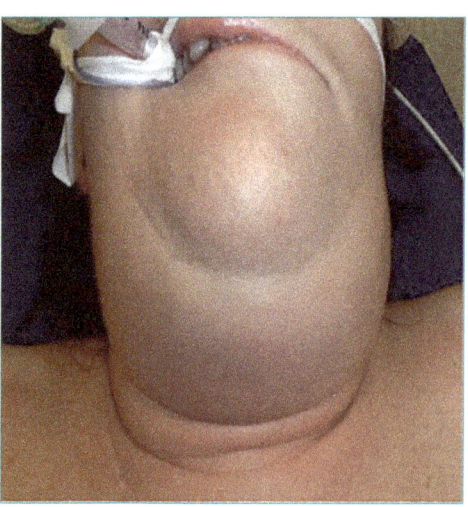

Figure 5.7: This patient presented with bilateral submandibular and submental collections. This is called 'Ludwig's angina'. This poses an immediate threat to the airway and requires urgent surgical and anaesthetic intervention. Picture courtesy of Mr. Madan Ethunandan

With experience, you will come to appreciate what needs a referral in urgently and what can be managed in an outpatient setting. (This is the value of seeing lots of patients in OMFS placements.)

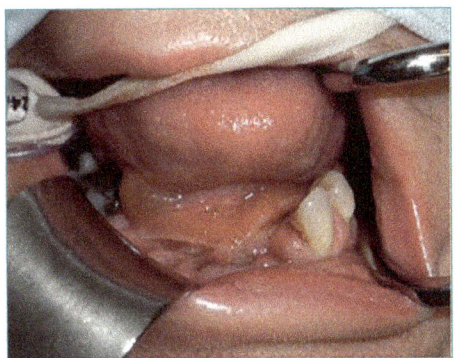

Figure 5.8: In Ludwig's angina, the patient presents with a 'raised floor of mouth', with the tongue pushed up. They can also have dysphonia or altered voice and difficulty swallowing their own saliva. Picture courtesy of Mr. Madan Ethunandan

Viral infections such as paramyxovirus can cause bilateral facial swelling, often seen in children and known as mumps. Other infectious sources of cervical lymphadenopathy include TB, EBV (glandular fever) and HIV, to name but a few.

5.2.2 CONGENITAL

A number of congenital masses are found in the head and neck region which, whilst they often present in children, it is not uncommon to first identify in adult patients. For some adults, they will only become a problem via an incidental finding or when they become infected.

Epidermoid cysts – These are also commonly known as 'sebaceous cysts'. They are caused by entrapment of embryonic-derived ectodermal tissues within the dermis. This can be because of trauma or due to obstructed sebaceous glands (so in these cases they are not technically speaking 'congenital'). Infected epidermoid cysts are common presentations to primary care. The overlying skin is erythematous and there is an associated swelling. Close examination reveals a 'punctum'. These should be treated in the first instance with oral antibiotics and/or drainage of any collections under LA. Following this, they can be formally excised in an outpatient setting once the infection/inflammation has resolved.

Dermoid cysts – Very much like epidermoid cysts, dermoid cysts arise from entrapment of ectoderm during fusion of embryologic lines. Characteristically, however, they differ from epidermoid cysts in that they contain dermal appendages – for example, hair follicles and sebaceous glands. Unlike epidermoid cysts, due to lines of fusion they are often found in the midline and paramedian regions, such as the midline of the neck and peri-orbital regions. These are again treated by surgical excision.

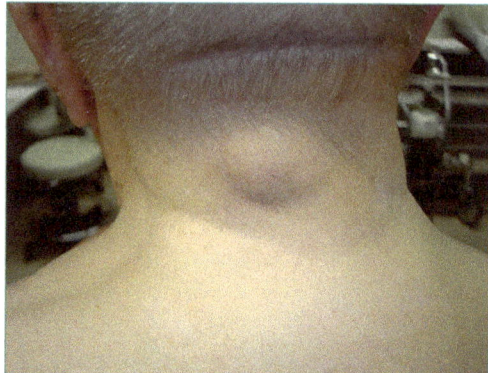

Figure 5.9: This patient presented with a mass in the nape of the neck. Notice a black mark in the centre of the lesion. This was a punctum. Picture courtesy of Mr. Stephen Walsh

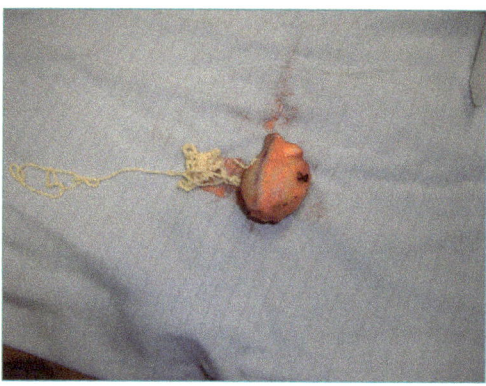

Figure 5.10: These are excised with an ellipse of skin enclosing the punctum. Here the surgeon has 'burst' the cyst to show the keratin found within the cyst cavity. Picture courtesy of Mr. Stephen Walsh

Thyroglossal cysts – The thyroid gland originally develops in the foramen caecum, found at the junction between the anterior two-thirds and posterior one-third of the tongue. The developing thyroid gland descends via the thyroglossal duct, a tubular structure passing anterior to the hyoid bone, prior to arriving in its final position in the anterior neck. The thyroglossal duct normally disintegrates following the migration of the thyroid gland. Failure of this results in a persistent thyroglossal duct on which cystic change can occur. Thyroglossal duct cysts commonly occur in the first two decades. They most commonly present with a midline swelling that can occur anywhere along the path of descent of the thyroid gland, though the bulk of them occur below the level of the hyoid bone. Notably, to distinguish thyroglossal duct cysts from other midline masses in the neck, ask the patient to protrude their tongue – this will cause upward movement, as they are almost always connected to the hyoid bone. Cross-sectional imaging and ultrasound-guided fine-needle aspiration cytology (FNAC) can aid diagnosis.

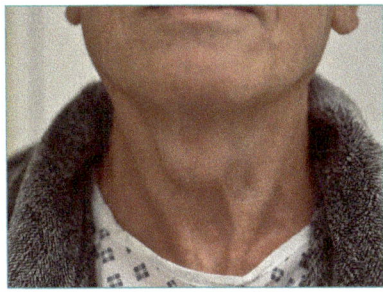
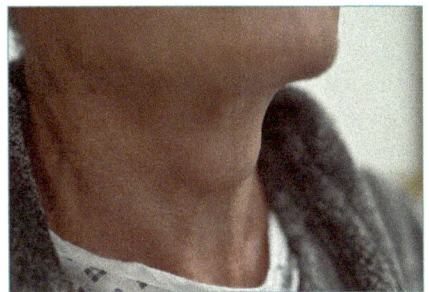

Figures 5.11 & 5.12: This patient presented with a midline neck mass. Pictures courtesy of Professor P. Brennan

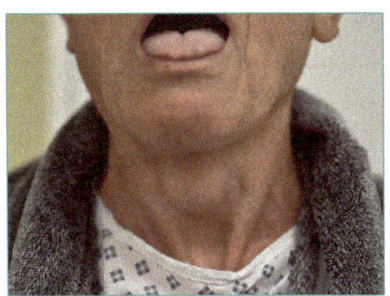

Figure 5.13: When asking the patient to protrude the tongue, the mass moved up the neck. This is in keeping with a thyroglossal cyst, as they are often attached to the hyoid bone. Picture courtesy of Professor P. Brennan

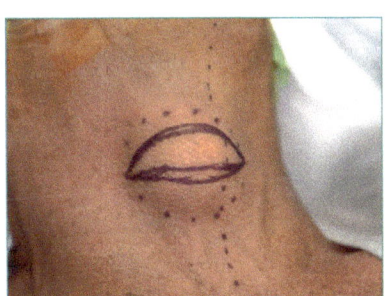
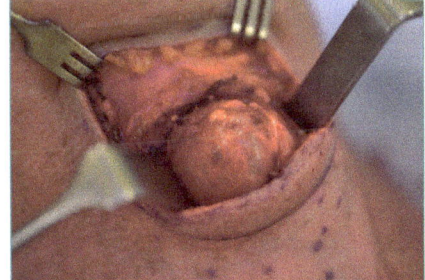
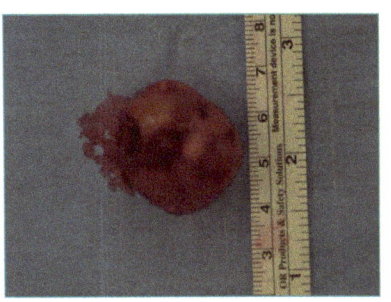

Figures 5.14, 5.15 & 5.16: Thyroglossal cysts are removed in a procedure called a 'Sistrunk procedure'. This requires excision of the cyst and duct but also part of the hyoid bone in order to prevent recurrence. Pictures courtesy of Professor P. Brennan

Management requires en-bloc excision of the thyroglossal cyst and tract, and some surgeons also remove the central part of the hyoid bone, to which it is commonly attached. This is called a 'Sistrunk procedure'. Failure to completely excise the duct can lead to recurrence and, very rarely, malignant change.

Branchial cyst – You may recall from embryology that from weeks three to eight in intra-uterine life, there are five pairs of branchial arches. These give rise to the major structures of the head and neck. The arches give rise to a number of branchial clefts, which are ectoderm lined and branchial, or pharyngeal pouches, which are endoderm lined. The mesoderm of the second branchial arch proliferates until it overlaps the third and fourth arches, leaving only a small ectoderm-lined sinus, known as the cervical sinus. This normally disappears with time; however, failure to involute or the persistence of cleft epithelia can result in branchial cysts, fistulae or sinuses. These present, most commonly, as neck swellings located along the anterior border of the sternocleidomastoid muscle, most commonly in the submandibular space; however, they can form anywhere from the parotid gland to the supraclavicular region. Third- and fourth-branchial-arch cysts are incredibly uncommon. They usually present as a soft, painless mass, but can become secondarily infected and are then tense with signs of inflammation.

When an adult over the age of 35–40 years presents with a potential branchial cyst (most present much earlier in life), it is important to exclude the possibility that the mass could be metastatic carcinoma within cystic cervical lymph nodes, most notably from the tonsils and oropharynx, or even malignant change in a branchial cyst. Where there is diagnostic uncertainty, cross-sectional imaging and/or ultrasound-guided fine-needle aspiration cytology (FNAC) can help delineate the cause. Management is in the form of surgical excision, and there is a fairly low rate of recurrence. Again, where there is any diagnostic uncertainty regarding potential malignant cause, they should be treated as malignant until proven otherwise.

Vascular malformations – The head and neck are an extremely vascular part of the body. As such, arteriovenous, capillary and lymphatic anomalies are reasonably common, either in isolation or as part of a systemic process or syndrome. Commonly, these lesions are investigated with ultrasound, MRI and/or CT. It is important to rule out any intracranial extension (which, if present, may put the patient at risk of catastrophic spontaneous intracranial haemorrhage). Treatment depends on cause: some lesions respond to beta-blockers (propranolol), whereas others may require cryotherapy, interventional radiology or even surgical removal. Our role as OMFS surgeons can be to help manage and support the airway if there is compromise and significant intra-oral extension associated with bleeding.

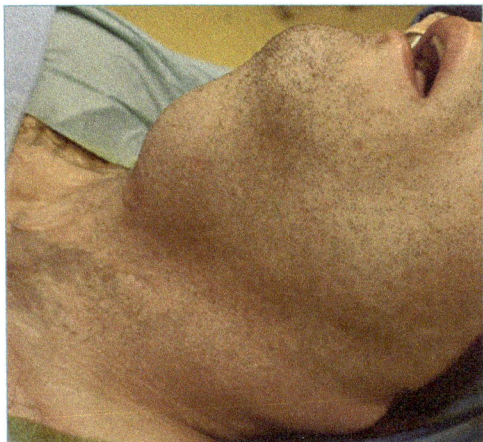

Figure 5.17: This gentleman presented with a submental swelling. Investigations including ultrasound and MRI revealed this to be an arteriovenous malformation. Picture courtesy of Mr. Madan Ethunandan

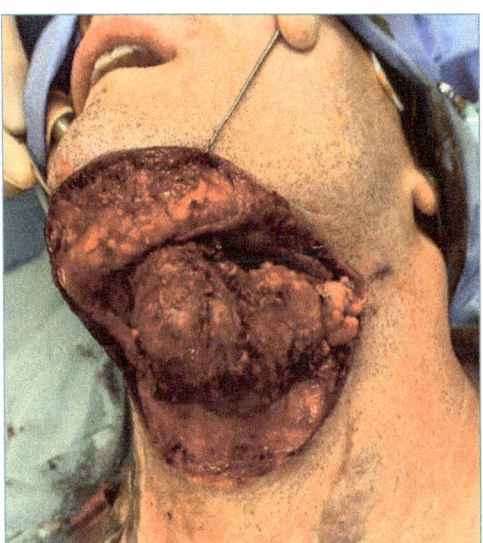

Figure 5.18: Following preoperative CT-guided embolisation, the malformation was surgically removed. Picture courtesy of Mr. Madan Ethunandan

5.2.3 NEOPLASTIC

Given that 300 of the total number of 800 or so lymph nodes are found in the head and neck, lymphoma often presents in the first instance as a neck mass. These are typically rubbery in consistency and usually multiple. Always ask patients about systemic symptoms such as loss of weight, night sweating and fever (also known as 'B symptoms'). Lymphoma is managed by haematologist but OMFS and ENT often help make the diagnosis, using US-guided core biopsies or even lymph-node biopsies in some cases.

A palpable malignant lymph node from a primary tumour in the head and neck is classically described as being hard or firm, progressing to a fixed mass with an irregular edge, and being larger than 1cm. This is due to the irregular growth of the cancer within the node and possible spread beyond its capsule into the adjacent tissue. In contrast, a reactive lymph node (secondary to infection/inflammation) exhibits hyperplasia of normal lymphoid tissue and is therefore contained within its capsule and presents as a firm but well-defined and mobile mass. A reactive lymph node will appear acutely and resolve as the infection subsides (i.e. within three weeks), whereas a malignant lymph node will present as a progressively enlarging mass over weeks or months.

It may be very difficult or impossible to discern between a reactive and neoplastic neck node. High suspicion for malignancy would warrant an USS with or without fine-needle aspiration cytology (FNAC). In cases of low suspicion, reassessment in two-to-three weeks is reasonable, with an USS if the node is still present.

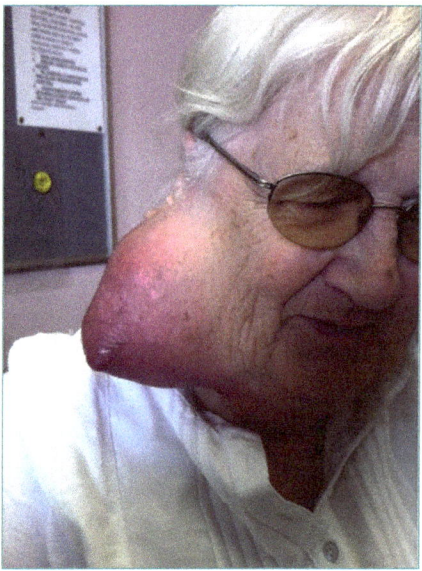

Figure 5.19: This lady presented with an extensive mass in the right neck/tail of parotid region. Picture courtesy of Professor P. Brennan

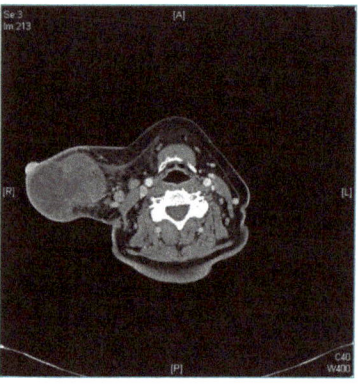

Figure 5.20: Cross-sectional imaging can be of huge diagnostic use. In this case, a CT with contrast was used to delineate the mass and give useful information of nearby major structures. Picture courtesy of Professor P. Brennan

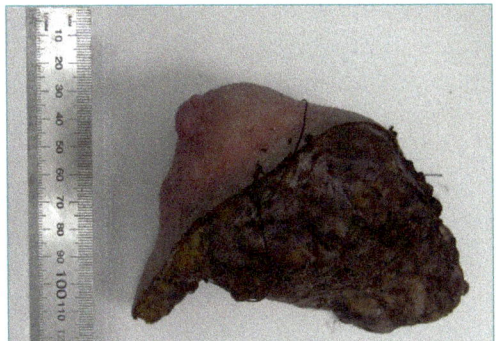

Figure 5.21: The mass excised. Picture courtesy of Professor P. Brennan

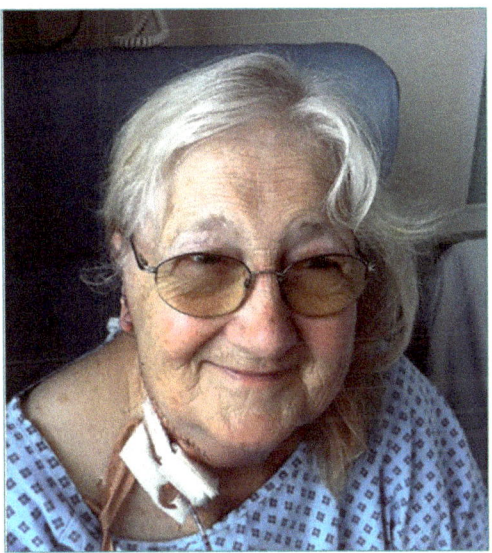

Figure 5.22: The postoperative result. Note that despite its proximity to the facial nerve, no branches or indeed the trunk were damaged. The patient had a House–Brackmann score of 1! Picture courtesy of Professor P. Brennan

There are many other causes of neck lumps but these are outside the scope of this book. The main thing is not to get overwhelmed, but to break things down into inflammatory, non-inflammatory, congenital and neoplastic (which can be primary or secondary) for starters!

Thyroid Masses

Patients presenting with a mass in the midline of the neck are an all-too-common referral to the neck-lump clinic (thyroglossal cyst has already been discussed above). While ENT and general surgeons have historically managed diseases of the thyroid that require surgery, increasingly OMFS are also operating on these fascinating lesions.

Fortunately, the overwhelming majority of solitary thyroid masses are benign. As with any suspected thyroid condition, a targeted history concerning signs of hyper- and hypothyroidism should be elicited, alongside questioning on dysphonia, stridor and dysphagia. A comprehensive neck examination should be performed, but one should also look for other features of extra-glandular disease manifestations.

Assessment can also involve blood tests, which are often done as part of routine assessment of any suspected thyroid lump. These include:

- TSH
- T3 Levels
- T4 Levels
- Antithyroid Peroxidase screen
- Antithyroglobulin screen.

In the first instance, ultrasound-guided fine-needle aspiration cytology (FNAC) can be hugely useful in arriving at a diagnosis. The use of radioisotope scanning can help differentiate between 'hot' and 'cold' nodules, and cross-sectional imaging such as CT and MRI can be used when assessing for metastatic disease.

Thyroid goitre ('goitre' means thyroid swelling) – Most enlargements of the thyroid gland are non-toxic goitres. This is compensatory hyperplasia of the gland as a consequence of persistent stimulation of TSH receptors. This may be due to increased physiological demand – for example, during pregnancy. It may, however, be secondary to iodine deficiency, which is oddly quite common, or Grave's disease. If non-toxic, they can be managed by mere active surveillance.

There are four main types of thyroid malignancy you need to be aware of, and often by attending a thyroid MDT (multidisciplinary team meeting) you will see multiple patients discussed and get a flavour of the assessment and investigations which drive their definitive management.

1. *Papillary carcinoma*
   Associated with a good prognosis, these can be managed with a lobectomy, total thyroidectomy and selective neck dissection if there are concerns about nodal involvement. Postoperatively, these patients are given life-long thyroxine to suppress their TSH levels, which are thought to be a causative factor.
2. *Follicular carcinoma*
   These are often a diagnostic challenge and patients often undergo a diagnostic hemithyroidectomy, which may then need to be completed

once formally reviewed. Follicular carcinoma spreads via the hematogenous route, so there is no need for elective neck dissection. However, life-long thyroxine supplementation is required.

3. *Medullary carcinoma*

   This arises from parafollicular cells and may be hereditary, being associated with multiple endocrine neoplasia (MEN) syndrome. These are treated with total thyroidectomy and neck dissection where required; however, unlike both papillary and follicular, medullary carcinoma is not sensitive to radioiodine or thyroxine.

4. *Anaplastic carcinoma*

   This is the rarest form and the most aggressive. Given its aggressive nature and often late presentation, this is often managed palliatively.

There are also parathyroid tumours (which often cause hypercalcaemia) but they do not often present as neck lumps, and are diagnosed on blood tests and nuclear medicine scans and are beyond the remit of this book.

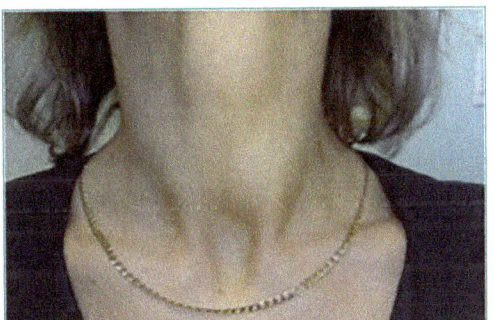

Figure 5.23: This lady presented with a midline neck mass which moved on swallowing, characteristic of thyroid masses. These can often be differentiated from thyroglossal cysts, which classically move 'up' with tongue protrusion. Picture courtesy of Mr. Stephen Walsh

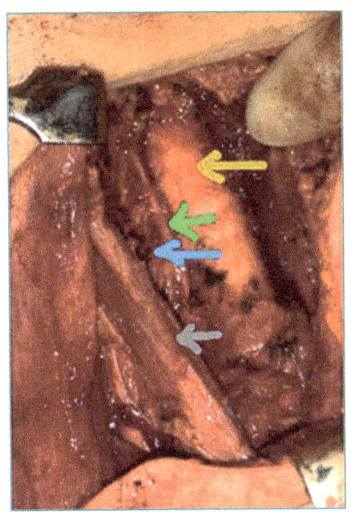

Figure 5.24: This is an intra-operative picture showing the number of structures closely related to the thyroid gland. Note that running in between the trachea (yellow arrow) and oesophagus (blue arrow) is the recurrent laryngeal nerve (green arrow). Picture courtesy of Mr. P. Alam

CHAPTER 6: FRONTAL BONE, CRANIUM AND ORBITS

6.1 INTRODUCTION

The frontal bone makes up the forehead and forms the anterior aspect of the cranium. There are key vital structures in this region, namely the brain and the orbits, as well as air-filled sinuses and spaces, soft-tissue structures (muscles and ducts), nerves, fat and skin. Importantly, abnormalities of the various structures within this region can present throughout life, from neonates to the very elderly.

6.2 ANATOMY

A brief understanding of some of the key anatomical structures will help you make sense of the pathology we encounter in this region. Starting deep, of course, is the brain, separated anteriorly from the outside world and orbits by the frontal bone. Within the frontal bone is the frontal sinus – an air-filled cavity lined with respiratory epithelium. The function of the frontal sinus is to humidify and filter the air breathed in by the nose. It produces mucous, which is used to trap bacteria, dust particles and other pollutants, which in turn drain into the nasal cavity through the fronto-nasal duct.

The rest of the bony structure of the orbit is predominantly made up of the zygoma laterally and the maxilla inferiorly. The sphenoid bone importantly separates the orbit from the intracranial cavity, but allows several important structures (e.g. some cranial nerves) to pass through it into the orbit. The orbital cavity contains a number of important structures including the globe (eye) and optic nerve, the six extraocular muscles and orbital fat, which are suspended by a network of ligaments.

Importantly, the development of the bony structures of the forehead and anterior skull are related to the other bones of the skull and 'sutures' which separate them. The bones of the skull form like tectonic plates in geography: as the brain grows in early life, it pushes these flat bones apart at the suture lines and new bone develops in the space. Premature closure of these sutures leads to abnormal skull growth, leading to changes in the shape (and function) of the structures in this region.

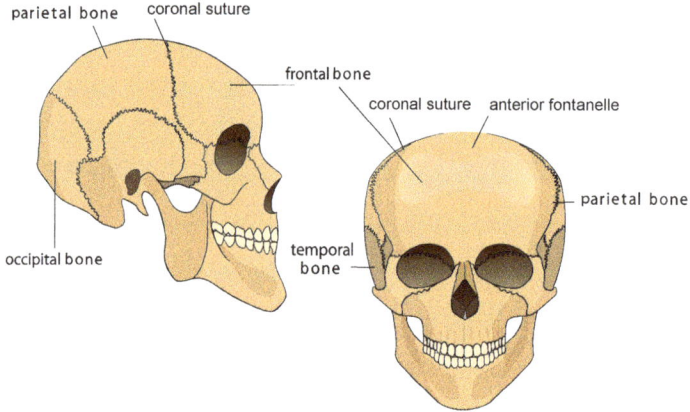

Figures 6.1 & 6.2: At birth the vault of the skull is created by a number of flat bones, separated by sutures. Where two or more sutures meet are fontanelles. Premature closure of these sutures and fontanelles can result in impaired craniofacial development.

Covering the bone is a layer of periosteum and muscle. The main muscle of the forehead is the frontalis muscle, which thins at its superior aspect, forming an aponeurotic (tendonous) layer in the scalp, which then envelops the occipital muscle posteriorly. This layer also continues inferiorly and links to the other muscles of facial expression. To the lateral side of the forehead is the temporalis muscle, a fan-shaped muscle on the sides of the head, the margin of which you can feel if you clench your teeth and palpate the lateral aspect of your forehead. This lateral aspect of the forehead is an important area, because here the temporal branch of the facial nerve runs very superficially. As a result, it is prone to injury in this area, via a number of pathological or iatrogenic mechanisms.

Other important nerves and vessels in the area are placed supero-medially around the orbit – in particular, the supratrochlear artery, which supplies the skin over the paramedian forehead, and which becomes very useful in facial reconstruction when creating a pedicled 'paramedian forehead flap' (for reconstructing the tip of the nose, for example). See section 7.6 for examples of how this is done.

6.2.1 SURGICAL ACCESS

The scalp has a fantastic blood supply, so bleeding from incisions and wounds can be dramatic. Using coronally orientated incisions, scars can be hidden

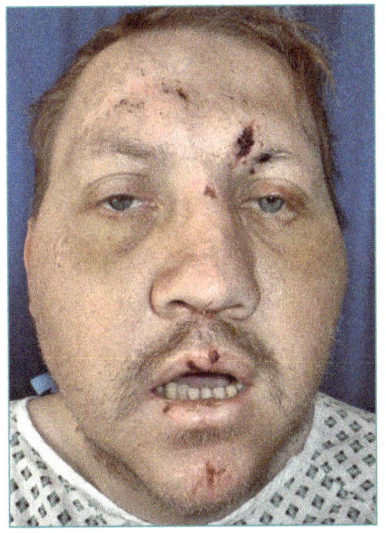

Figure 6.3: This gentleman presented with multiple fractures to the facial skeleton. This is often described as 'pan-facial fractures'. Picture courtesy of Mr. Madan Ethunandan

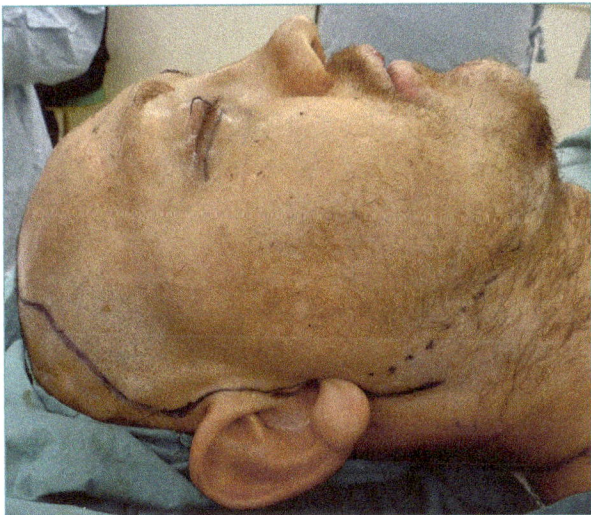

Figure 6.4: Due to its excellent vascularity, an incision can be placed in the hair-bearing regions of the scalp and the face 'peeled down' to expose the fractures using a top-to-bottom approach. This is called a 'coronal flap'. The patient was shaved moments before surgery to reduce the potential for infection. Picture courtesy of Mr. Madan Ethunandan

posteriorly, in the hair-bearing areas, thereby avoiding important soft-tissue structures and unsightly scars. The scalp can then be peeled forward and backward, allowing access to the bones of the skull. Furthermore, an in-depth knowledge of the different layers through which the temporal branch of the facial nerve runs allows us to expose the forehead, temple region, orbit and zygomatic arch, while minimising any risks to the facial nerve itself. Once these bony structures are exposed, the underlying pathology can be addressed in whatever form is required.

6.3 TRAUMATIC INJURIES TO THE FRONTAL BONE

Fractures to the frontal bone, caused by blows to the forehead, are important for two reasons. Firstly, because of the prominence of the forehead and superior orbital rim on the face, and the relatively thin overlying cutaneous tissues, any damage to this area can leave marked aesthetic deformities. However, of greater concern is any involvement of the posterior table (the posterior wall of the sinus, closest to the brain) of the frontal sinus, as this can provide a pathway for infection to spread directly into the anterior cranial fossa and to the brain itself.

Such injuries disrupt the underlying dura (one of the membranes which covers the brain). This can result in the leaking of cerebrospinal fluid (CSF), which leaks through the fracture, into the frontal sinus, through the fronto-nasal duct and then presents as CSF rhinorrhoea – which is the term used to describe leaking of clear straw-coloured fluid from the nose. It is of course difficult to differentiate CSF rhinorrhoea from typical nasal discharge in the trauma setting, as both appear as clear fluids. If this happens, a sample can be sent to the lab, where electrophoresis can confirm the presence of β2 transferrin, a protein which is found exclusively in the CSF.

A CT scan is the most helpful radiological investigation for trauma to this region and allows us to analyse in detail the site and the extent of the fracture, which helps to determine the nature of the surgical procedure required. Importantly, with these injuries, the aim of management is to ensure that the fractured frontal sinus does not lead to infection or inflammation around

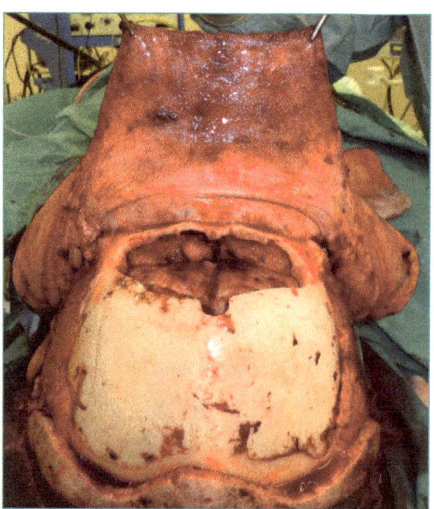

Figure 6.5: As part of the pan-facial fractures, the patient presented with a depressed frontal bone fracture. A coronal flap was raised to allow access to the frontal bone and zygomatic arches. In this picture you can see into the frontal sinus. The surgeon is lifting the periosteum of the skull, otherwise known as the pericranium, which can be used to seal the frontal sinus from nasal passages. Picture courtesy of Mr. Madan Ethunandan

the brain, and to reconstruct the bony contour appropriately. Sometimes, surgical corrections require full coronal access, with craniotomies. However, in less-significant injuries, fractures can be reduced and fixed endoscopically. Sometimes, the bony contour can even be camouflaged using other techniques such as fat grafting.

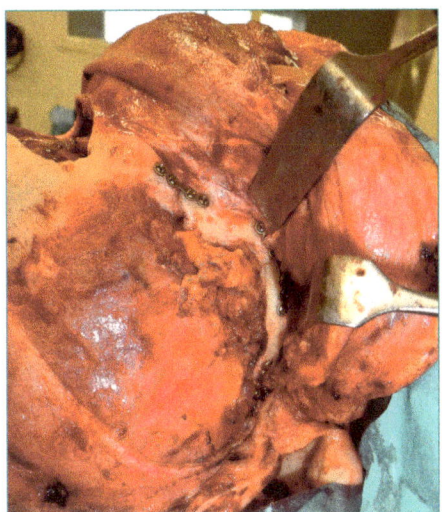

Figure 6.6: *The coronal flap also allows access to the supra-orbital rim and the arch of the zygoma. Here you can see where the surgeon has isolated these regions, reduced the underlying fractured bones and immobilised the bones in their correct positions with plates and screws. Picture courtesy of Mr. Madan Ethunandan*

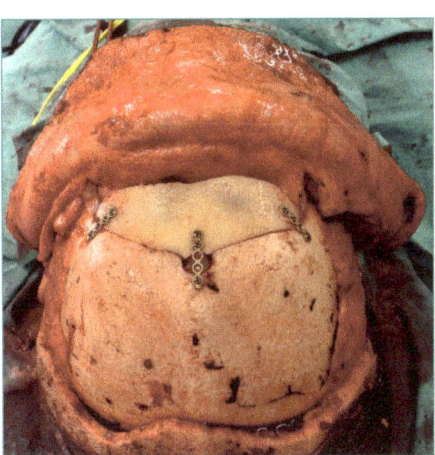

Figure 6.7: *Following this, the patient's frontal bone was placed into the correct position and immobilised or 'fixed' in this position with plates and screws. Picture courtesy of Mr. Madan Ethunandan*

6.4 ORBITAL FRACTURES

Directly inferior to the forehead are the orbits. Medial to them is the nose, inferiorly the maxilla, and inferolateral are the cheek prominences of the zygoma. There are some natural weak points where the continuity of the orbital skeleton can be disrupted. Firstly, the floor of the orbit (also the roof of the maxillary sinus) is egg-shell thin. So too is the medial wall, formed by the delicate lacrimal and ethmoid bones (described as 'lamina papyracea' – Latin for 'paper thin'). These areas can often crumble after a blow to the region. There are other areas around the orbit which can also fracture, but we will discuss those a little later.

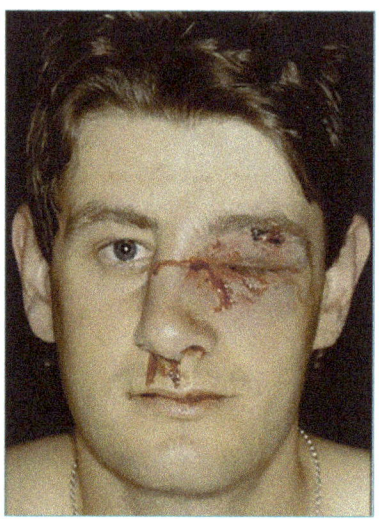

Figure 6.8: This young man has been assaulted. Initial assessment of his face suggests nasal bone fractures, as his nose is clearly deviating to the right. However, it is essential to open the left eye to assess for any underlying orbital trauma. Picture courtesy of Mr. Graham Bounds

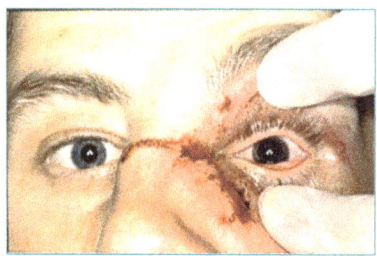

Figure 6.9: After opening the eye, the pupils are assessed for direct and consensual light responses. Visual acuity can be crudely assessed prior to a more detailed examination for disrupted eyeball movement or diplopia. Picture courtesy of Mr. Graham Bounds

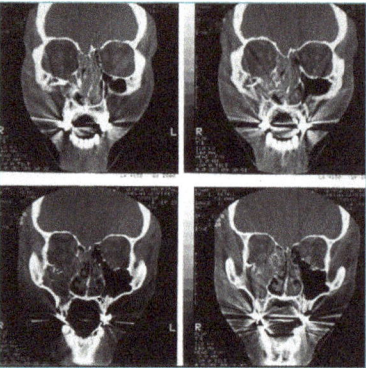

Figure 6.10: Whilst plain film x-rays can be of use, CT scans are the gold standard for assessment for orbital fractures. Here are images of a right orbital floor and medial wall fracture. Note how clear (black) the left maxillary sinus is. The right is full of fluid (grey) and you can see part of the floor of the right orbit pushed into the sinus. Picture courtesy of Mr. Graham Bounds

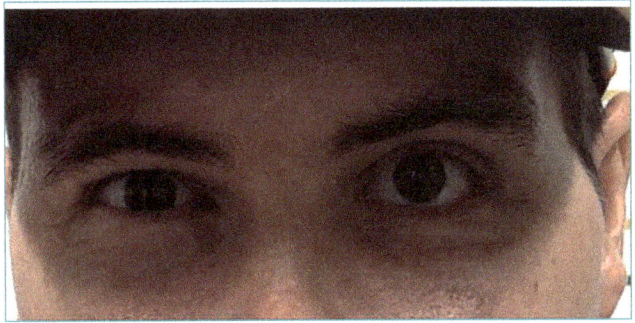

Figure 6.11: Notice how the right eye looks lower than the left. The best way to assess this is to draw an imaginary line between the two pupils. The right pupil is below this line. This is called 'hypoglobus'. Picture courtesy of Miss Nabeela Ahmed

It is unsurprising that a patient who has suffered a blow to the orbital region will present with swelling and peri-orbital bruising. In the case of a fracture to the floor of the orbit, sometimes, the fat, or even the inferior rectus muscle, can get trapped in the fracture line, leading to a restriction in upward gaze. This may resolve as the swelling settles. However, what happens after the swelling resolves becomes most important in managing these patients – and these sequelae relate to orbital volume. By this, we mean that fractures to those bones mentioned above lead to an increase in orbital volume. In patients with more significant bony defects, this ultimately leads to a change in the position of the globe, where it either sinks backwards into the orbit (enophthalmos) or drops down (hypoglobus).

To stop this from happening, we often reconstruct these areas with prefabricated orbital titanium meshes, which support the globe in its normal position and stop it from sinking backwards and downwards. One of the commonest ways these are placed is via a trans-conjunctival approach, where the cut (and therefore scar) is hidden in the inner aspect of the lower eyelid. Here, we rely on a detailed appreciation of eyelid anatomy to carefully evert the lower lid, incise the conjunctiva, dissect our way toward the orbital rim before incising the periosteum. This allows us to gently lift the globe without damage, to explore the orbital floor and, if needed, the medial wall, to position the implant. This can often be done without leaving an external scar.

Another interesting thought about orbital-floor fractures relates to the differences between adult and paediatric bone characteristics. You will probably recall how adult bones tend to be more brittle, while those of children are more elastic and spring like. While adult bones tend to fracture (as

108 ORAL AND MAXILLOFACIAL SURGERY

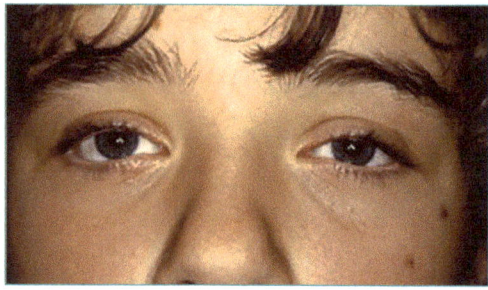

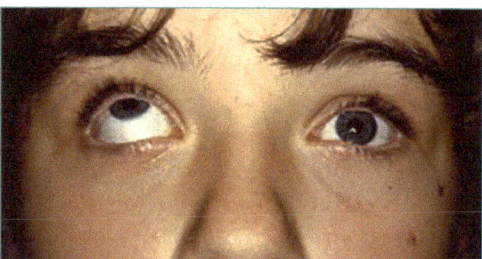

Figures 6.12 & 6.13: This young man on first inspection looks absolutely normal. There is no subconjunctival haemorrhage or hypoglobus. However, on moving the eye there is clear restriction of the left eye on upward gaze. This is due to muscle entrapment. This is called 'white-eye orbital-floor fracture' and mainly occurs in children. Picture courtesy of Mr. Graham Bounds

described above), in children who suffer a blow to the orbital region, the bones of the orbital floor can partially break, distort and then spring back into place. In doing so, they trap the soft tissues in the fracture line. This entrapment evokes an oculo-cardiac reflex – leading to nausea, vomiting and bradycardia. Unlike the situation above, this warrants immediate attention, involving release of the tissues to prevent life-altering morbidity.

6.5 ORBITAL COMPARTMENT SYNDROME

As mentioned above, the orbit is a bony cavity with no ability to expand. The contents of the cavity are kept in place by a network of tight ligaments anteriorly. As a result, any swelling behind the eye will increase the intra-orbital pressure and compress the important neurovascular structures (optic nerve and retinal artery) there. Such a swelling is typically caused by traumatic injury, but can also be caused by neoplastic or other inflammatory processes. Bleeding behind the eye caused by trauma can also lead to this increase in intra-orbital pressure and compression. If because of bleeding this is termed a 'retrobulbar haemorrhage' or if because of swelling only an 'orbital compartment syndrome'. This is a surgical emergency as if untreated will result in blindness of the affected eye.

The rise in intra-orbital pressure leads to disproportionate pain behind the eye, reduced and painful eye movements (ophthalmoplegia), proptosis (where

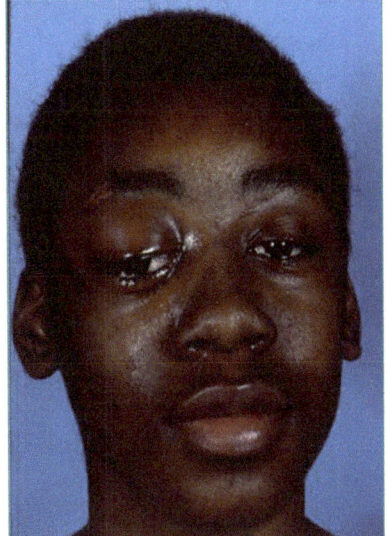 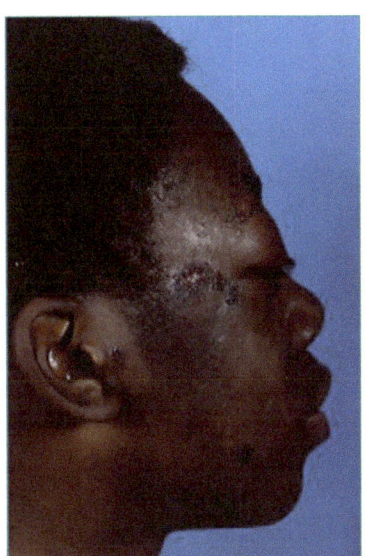

Figures 6.14 & 6.15: This young man presented with excruciating pain from the right orbital region. Note how pushed forward his eye is. This is proptosis. He also had a progressively dilated pupil. This was retrobulbar haemorrhage and needed urgent medical and surgical intervention. Pictures courtesy of Mr. G. Bounds

the eye appears pushed out of the socket), a tense globe and reduced visual acuity.

This is a sight-threatening emergency and urgent action needs to be taken to avoid permanent blindness. This takes the form of a surgical decompression, where the lateral canthus, which holds the lateral aspects of the upper and lower eyelid to the lateral orbital wall, is cut to allow the pressure behind the eye to be released. Members of the maxillofacial emergency team are taught how to do this as a sight-saving procedure.

6.6 CRANIOFACIAL SURGERY

Another set of pathologies are those that relate to the abnormal development of the bony structures and soft-tissue structures of the face. These are often related to the premature or incomplete fusion of various facial structures during embryonic development.

When cranial sutures fuse prematurely, it is called 'craniosynostosis'. This restricts the growth of the cranial vault at the suture line, and instead the skull grows in different directions to accommodate the developing brain. Sometimes more than one suture is involved, and this may occur as part of a syndrome. Importantly, this premature fusion can impact the skull base and facial skeleton, leading not only to abnormally shaped skull vaults, but raised intracranial pressures, ocular problems and restricted midface growth with associated risks to the airway.

Managing these patients is complex, involving a multidisciplinary team (MDT) including not only OMFS, but also our allied surgical specialities – plastic surgery and neurosurgery – as well as paediatrics, speech and language therapy (SALT), and dietetics. Surgery, which is usually performed within the first year of life, often involves excision of the fused suture, but also cranial-vault remodelling. In other words, cuts are made in the bony skull to create space. The fragments are then either repositioned using resorbable (slowly dissolving) plates and screws, or they are moved more gradually through a process called 'distraction osteogenesis'.

6.7 SKIN CANCERS OF THE SCALP AND FOREHEAD

The scalp and forehead are very common areas to develop cutaneous (skin) malignancies. The commonest kinds of cancers are basal cell carcinomas (BCC) and squamous cell carcinomas (SCC). These cancers can be treated with radiotherapy, but more often require surgical excision. To do so safely requires a wide local excision where the cancers are removed with a 4–6mm margin of normal-looking skin around the tumour.

Although these numbers sound small, on the forehead and scalp they can lead to considerably sized defects. It is often difficult to close these defects primarily (by directly opposing the skin edges), and as such, it is common to close these areas using local skin flaps, which are essentially a way of utilising the laxity in nearby skin to close the defect in such a way that limits the tension across the healing scar.

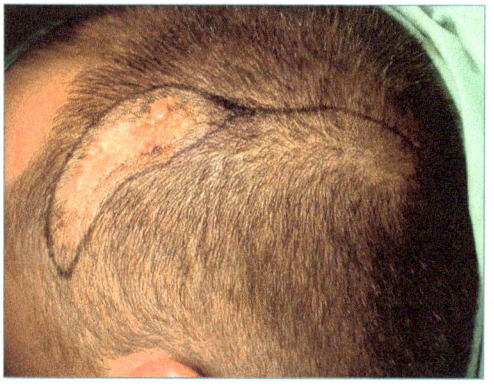

Figure 6.16: This gentleman presented with a lesion in the hair-bearing region of the scalp. Picture courtesy of Professor P. Brennan

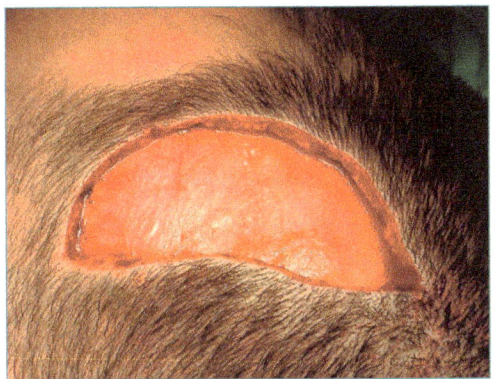

Figure 6.17: Following excision of the lesion, he was left with a considerable defect. Picture courtesy of Professor P. Brennan

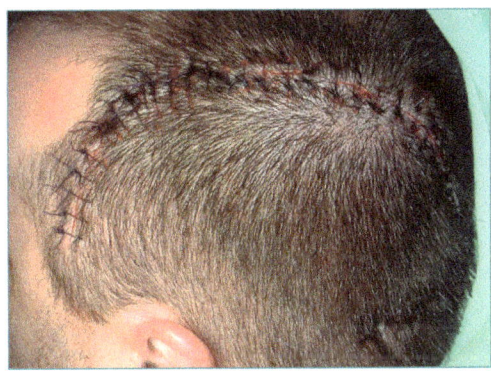

Figure 6.18: Here a local flap was used and rotated into the defect. This allowed for 'stretching' of the adjacent skin into the defect, leaving the patient with only a linear scar that will be hidden by his hair. Picture courtesy of Professor P. Brennan

Defects on the forehead can cause particular aesthetic compromise and patients are often worried about scarring. To minimise this, excision (and local flap reconstruction) is done in such a way that best camouflages the scars, often making use of the horizontal relaxed skin tension lines – indicated by the skin creases left by the wrinkles in the forehead. This leads to a sideways 'H'-shaped scar, which leaves the best possible scar.

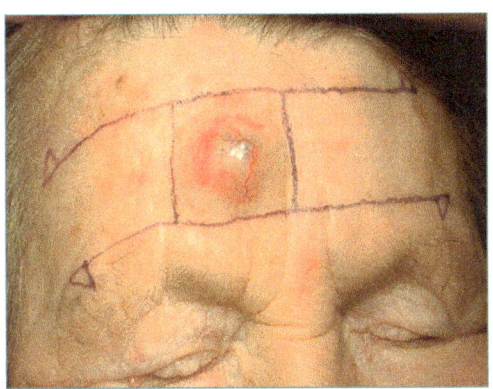

Figure 6.19: This elderly lady presented with a cutaneous malignancy in the midline of the forehead. Picture courtesy of Professor P. Brennan

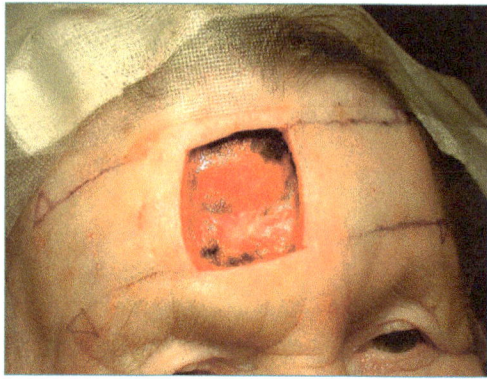

Figure 6.20: In order to increase the chance of complete clearance of the tumour, a margin of 'normal' tissue is excised all around the tumour. This left a considerable defect that could not be closed by primary closure. Picture courtesy of Professor P. Brennan

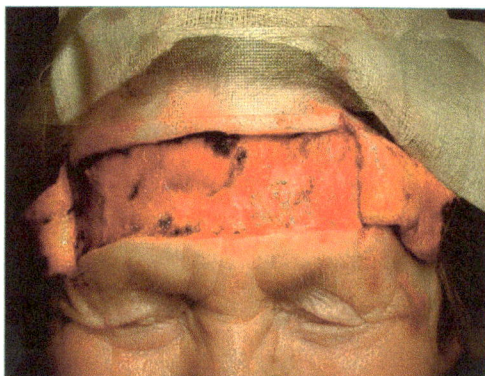

Figure 6.21: A local flap was used, where our knowledge of wrinkles or relaxed skin tension lines allows us to recruit neighbouring skin into the defect whilst placing incisions in 'wrinkles'. Picture courtesy of Professor P. Brennan

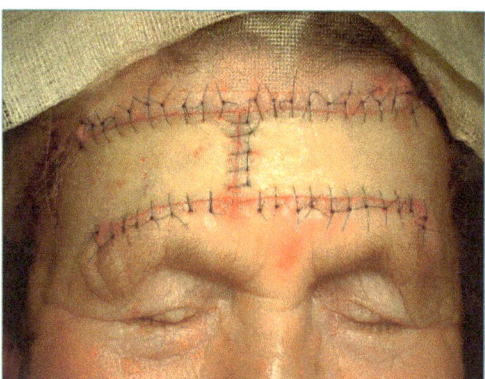

Figure 6.22: The finished result! With time, the incisions will look like wrinkle lines on the patient's forehead. Picture courtesy of Professor P. Brennan

In the hair-bearing area of the scalp, larger defects can also be covered by a skin graft. Biological scaffolds can also be used (for example, a porcine/bovine dermis substitute) which facilitate healing.

In this chapter, we hope to have guided you through some of the common problems that we encounter in the upper one-third of the face. As you will see throughout this book, problems can arise at multiple different levels or involve different tissues within the region – skin, muscle, nerves or bone. We hope you can also appreciate the range in age of patients that can be treated, from the paediatric neonate with a craniofacial deformity, through to the octogenarian with a cutaneous malignancy.

CHAPTER 7: NOSE AND SINUSES

7.1 INTRODUCTION

The air spaces in the facial region – namely the nasal cavity and the paranasal sinuses – are complex. Because of their complexity, we often find ourselves working closely with other surgical specialities – ENT (ear, nose and throat) surgeons, plastic surgeons, oculoplastic surgeons, neurosurgeons and ophthalmic surgeons, to name a few – to best manage the range of pathologies that arise in this region. In this chapter, we'll discuss how the oral and maxillofacial surgeon might encounter these pathologies.

7.2 ANATOMY

The nose connects the outside world to the nasopharynx. It aids breathing and our ability to smell. It has a rigid bony framework superiorly and a more flexible, cartilaginous framework inferiorly. Overlying this is a thin layer of muscle, subcutaneous fat and skin. The inside of the nose is divided into left and right nasal spaces by a cartilaginous nasal septum. On each lateral nasal wall are three invaginations (the inferior, middle and superior turbinates), which serve to increase the surface area of the mucosa that lines the inner surface of the nose. Between each turbinate is a space – a meatus – into which the paranasal sinuses drain. In addition, the nasolacrimal duct drains tears from the medial aspect of the eye into the nose.

There are four pairs of paranasal sinuses – the maxillary (which is our key concern in this chapter), the frontal (which you have met already in the previous chapter), the ethmoid and the sphenoid sinuses (which lie slightly deeper behind the nose). These sinuses are surrounded by thin, egg-shell-like bone. Their purpose is not yet fully clear, but many think they serve as a physiological crumple zone, dissipating the forces around the facial skeleton to avoid significant injuries to the vital structures (eyes and brain).

There is a small hole in the front of the maxillary sinus where the infra-orbital nerve emerges. This nerve is a branch of the trigeminal nerve, and runs directly underneath the orbital floor before emerging through the infra-orbital foramen. It supplies sensation to the cheek, lateral nose and upper teeth. When the nearby bones are fractured – for example, the roof of the maxillary sinus (or the orbital floor) – patients often report an altered sensation in the distribution of this nerve, as it has become stretched, bruised, swollen or cut.

7.3 FRACTURES

The nose has a prominent position on the face and so, like the mandible, it is prone to traumatic injury. Common causes of nasal bone fractures, indeed any facial bone fracture, are interpersonal violence, sports injuries and road-traffic accidents (RTAs). Sometimes patients present with isolated nasal bone fractures, but it is also common for patients to present to us with nasal fractures as part of more complex facial trauma. Here they can present alongside orbital wall fractures, zygomatic or maxillary fractures, or as part of more complicated naso-orbito-ethmoidal complex or midface fractures.

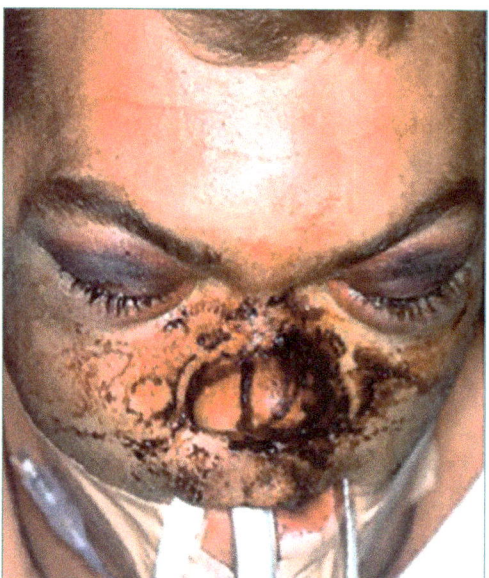

Figure 7.1: This patient presented with significant facial trauma. He had comminuted fractures of his nasal bones, but also involving his orbital and ethmoidal bones. These are commonly called 'naso-orbital-ethmoidal fractures' or 'NOE'. Picture courtesy of Mr. Andrew Sidebottom

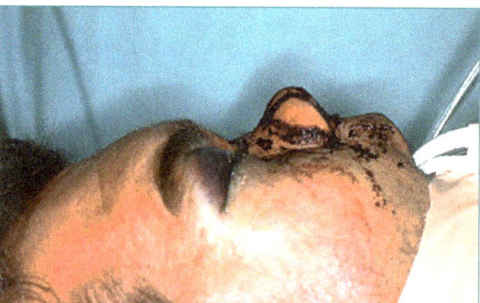

Figure 7.2: Notice from this side-on picture that you can really see how 'dished in' the bridge of the nose is. Such fractures can also cause separation of the medial canthi called 'telecanthus'. Picture courtesy of Mr. Andrew Sidebottom

Luckily, unlike the long bone fractures that orthopaedic surgeons might encounter, the physiological forces on the midface bones (such as the nasal bones, midface and zygoma) are distributed in different ways. Fractures of these bones will often heal by themselves (wherever they end up lying). As a result, not every fracture requires operative intervention, provided there is no significant visible deformity. Therefore, when patients suffer facial fractures, it is important for us to make an accurate assessment of exactly what the traumatic deformity looks like.

Due to the natural, and important, inflammatory response to any acute injury, post-traumatic swelling typically worsens over the first 48–72 hours. This makes it difficult to make an accurate assessment of any facial defect in the first few days after an injury. However, after that time, swelling begins to settle. As such, it is not uncommon for us to wait for 7–10 days after the actual injury to bones of the midface to make a decision about whether a fracture requires any operative intervention. Importantly, this time is not wasted! Aside from allowing the swelling to settle, because these fractures involve or are close to the orbit, this 10-day window is invaluable in allowing us to liaise with our ophthalmology colleagues to ensure there is no accompanying eye injury and arrange appropriate imaging.

Bones take several weeks to heal after they have been fractured. This leaves the oral and maxillofacial surgeon a window of time to correct these bony defects – to allow soft-tissue swelling to settle, but before the bones have started to remodel and heal. Therefore, when operative fixation is warranted, we aim to do this within three-to-four weeks; otherwise, the bone edges become sticky and more difficult to put back in the correct position.

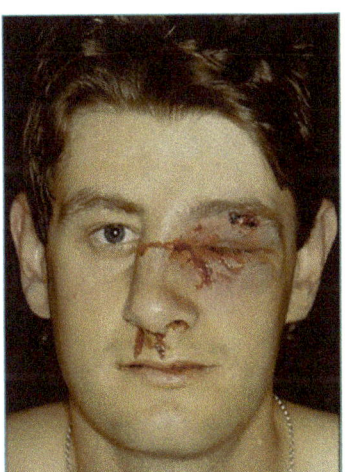

Figure 7.3: If this patient had no other injuries and only the obvious nasal bone fracture, he may well have been a candidate for 'closed reduction' or manipulation of nasal bones under anaesthesia. Picture courtesy of Mr. Graham Bounds

Following this, displaced nasal bone fractures are generally managed in a 'closed' fashion. Here, there is no incision and exposure of the bone itself. Instead, under general anaesthesia, the nasal bones are manipulated back into an appropriate position, and a small nasal splint is applied for several weeks to hold them in position.

In patients with more significant deformities, those with older injuries or those where a manipulation has not succeeded in appropriately realigning the nose, more complex procedures are required. This is because the traumatic injury has led to damage to the cartilaginous framework of the nose, or because the bony fragments of the nose have healed in an incorrect position and are no longer moveable by simple manipulation. Sometimes, the position of the cartilaginous framework needs to be corrected, which is called a 'septoplasty'. Here, the deformed cartilage of the nasal septum is removed, reshaped and repositioned. Occasionally, we borrow cartilage from elsewhere – for example, the costal cartilage of a rib or ear. Sometimes, the nasal bones need to be osteotomised (i.e. re-broken) and repositioned, in what is known as a 'rhinoplasty'. Sometimes both of these are required to correct the post-traumatic nasal defect – a septorhinoplasty.

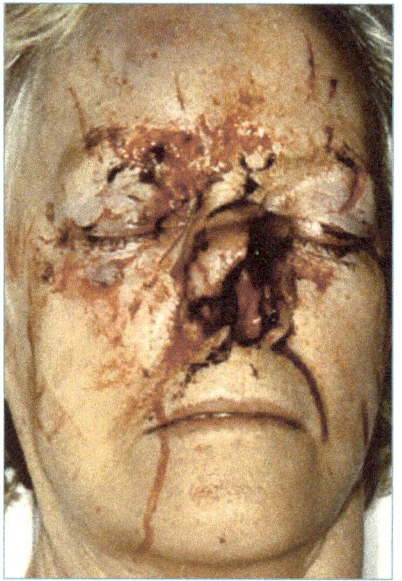 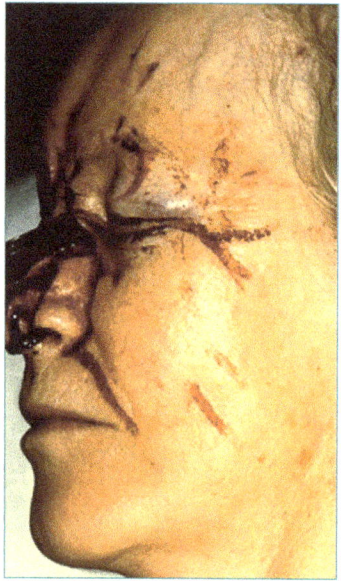

Figures 7.4 & 7.5: Due to the extent of the injuries sustained, this patient would have needed attention not only to the superficial structures, but also to rebuild the cartilaginous and bony skeleton of the nose. Pictures courtesy of Mr. G. Bounds

Patients with cleft lip and palate often require similar procedures because the growth, development and therefore shape of the nose have been highly disrupted. Similarly, in other craniofacial deformities, such as those encountered in section 3.3, when the upper jaw is moved around into its correct position, adjustments to the nasal septum and bones are often required to avoid disruption to nasal structures.

On either side of the nasal cavity are the maxillary sinuses. These air spaces are lined with respiratory epithelium and contained within relatively thin bone. Above the maxillary sinus is the floor of the orbit. You can feel the anterior wall just lateral to the nose, and might just be able to get to its posterolateral wall if you can get your finger anywhere beyond your upper wisdom teeth! As mentioned above, the maxillary sinus serves as a biological crumple zone – which means it often fractures during trauma to the face. As with the nose, sometimes these fractures are isolated to a single maxillary sinus wall, but often they involve one or more walls, or occur with other bony fractures.

Lateral to the maxillary sinus is the zygoma – the cheekbone. Like the nose, its prominence on the lateral aspect of the face leaves it prone to traumatic injury. The zygoma has a posterior extension, which forms an arch between the bones on the front of the head and those on the side of the head (aka the 'cheekbones'). This arch is a remarkable piece of anatomy that can be lifted with an instrument to effectively reposition the body of the zygoma when we repair fractures that involve the zygoma.

As you have seen throughout this book, oral and maxillofacial surgeons have unique and varied ways to access, reduce and fix facial bone fractures, and to minimise conspicuous scars. We are always trying to hide scars in areas that are not usually visible – for example, in the hairline, in the mouth, in the natural skin creases and even in the conjunctiva. We can do this because the face has a wonderfully rich blood supply, and we can pull and stretch the skin in a way that is sometimes the envy of surgeons who operate on other parts of the body.

7.4 BLEEDING

A patient with isolated nasal bleeding (epistaxis) tends to find their way to our ENT colleagues. However, it is important to realise that nosebleeds can also arise secondary to other facial injuries – in particular, when there are fractures that involve the maxillary sinuses or midface. We have already seen that the sinus is closely related to the nose – lying beside and connected to it. Therefore, when the maxillary sinus fills with blood, it can often overflow into the nose

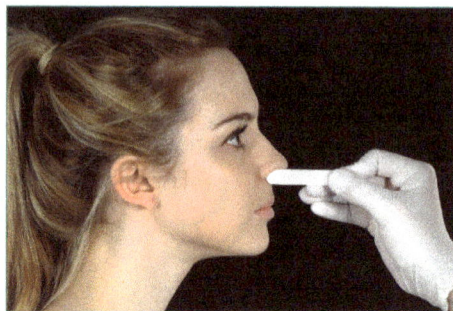

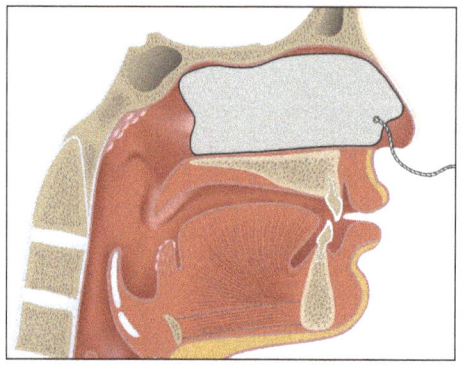

*Figure 7.6: Procedure for anterior nasal packing using a Merocel® **nasal** tampon. (a) Insertion of the tampon (note the angle of insertion) and (b) the tampon expanded within the nasal cavity.*

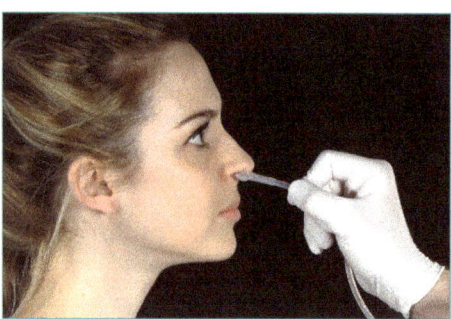

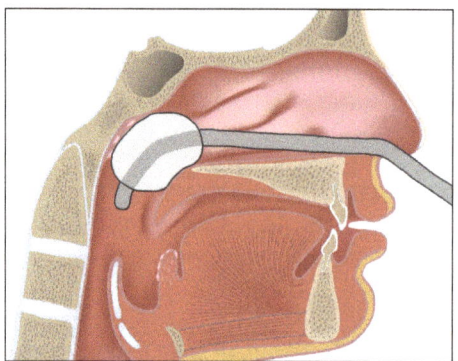

Figure 7.7: Procedure for posterior nasal packing using a Foley catheter. (a) Insertion of the catheter (note the angle of insertion) and (b) the catheter balloon expanded within the posterior nasal space.

and lead to bleeding through the nostril or posterior nose. This can happen with any midface trauma. To stop the bleeding, in the first instance, we can pack the nose (anteriorly and posteriorly).

Figures 7.6 and 7.7 show the method of both anterior and posterior nasal packing. The aim is to stop the bleeding by pressure or tamponade. However, sometimes this doesn't control the bleeding from a midface fracture because the edges of the fractured bones themselves continue to bleed. The way to stop this bleeding is to compress the bone edges, which we do indirectly with a bite block. Of course, once the acute bleeding has settled, these injuries may well require operative fixation under GA, where we can ensure the fractures are reduced and fixed in the correct place using a combination of miniplates, wires and braces.

Along similar lines, the presence of fluid in the maxillary sinus (particularly in a patient who has suffered an injury to the face) can also help support a diagnosis of a facial bone fracture. Noting the presence of fluid in the sinus has become an important part of analysing a facial bones radiograph.

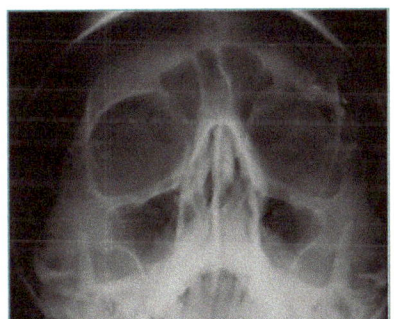

Figure 7.8: This is an occipitomental or 'facial view' radiograph. As you can see, this patient is actually post-surgery, having had their left supra-orbital rim fracture repaired with wiring. This x-ray shows that normally the maxillary sinuses are black. When looking for fractures of the midface, the sinuses can often fill with blood or herniated orbital contents. This would appear on an x-ray as grey contents within the sinus. Picture courtesy of Mr. Graham Bounds

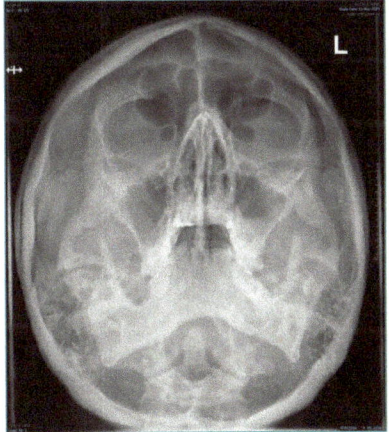

Figure 7.9: Facial bones showing an air/fluid level in the left maxillary sinus. This does not always correlate with a fracture of the midface – so imaging should be used to support clinical diagnosis, not replace it. Picture courtesy of Miss Nabeela Ahmed

7.5 DENTAL PATHOLOGY

Aside from being intimately related to the orbit above and the lateral nose to the side, the maxillary sinus is also closely related to the upper teeth – and in particular to the premolar and large molar teeth on either side.

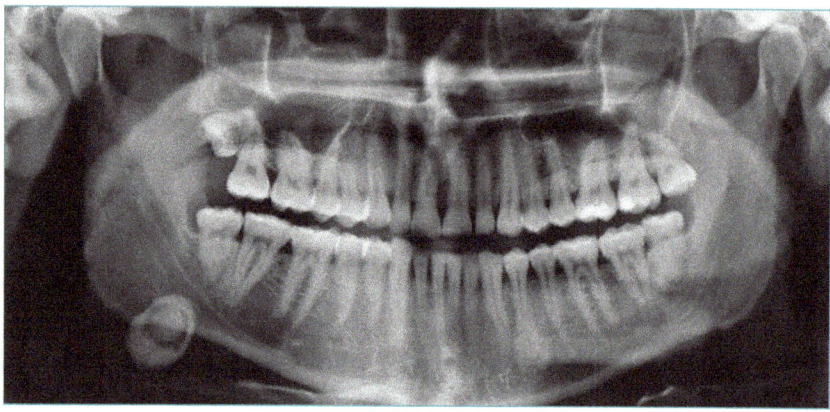

Figure 7.10: Whilst this OPG shows a right submandibular duct stone, it also shows the close proximity of the upper teeth to the maxillary sinuses. It is not uncommon for a root to be pushed into the sinuses when a dentist extracts it, or more commonly, for a hole to remain between the sinus and oral cavity. This is called an 'oroantral communication'. Picture courtesy of Mr. Stephen Walsh

This is important for a number of reasons. Problems with these teeth – such as acute or chronic dental infections – can lead to sinusitis-like symptoms; and conversely, sinus inflammation can lead to dental pain. Each can be mistaken for the other! Here, a thorough history and examination of the patient can help to differentiate between the two.

In addition, there are a number of cyst-like lesions that can arise from or around teeth and extend into the maxillary sinus. The most common cysts tend to arise from teeth that have had chronic infections, but there are many differentials. Occasionally, we might be required to retrieve a tooth root or dental filling material that has become displaced into the sinus! For upper first and second premolars in particular, there is a risk of pushing these teeth, or their roots, into the sinus during extraction procedures, due to the forces needed to remove them. In such cases, we may need to make a small cut in the mucosa of the upper arch, find the anterior wall of the sinus and make a small window in the maxillary bone to access whatever is inside. Due to the close proximity of the apices of upper posterior teeth to the sinus, there is also the risk of tearing the maxillary sinus lining when removing such teeth. This causes what we call an 'oroantral communication', where there is a direct communication between the mouth and the maxillary sinus. If large and left untreated, this can, over time, form an oroantral fistula. Patients may present following an extraction complaining of water extruding from their nose, or a funny taste of nasal discharge from the sinus in their mouth! Small defects will often resolve spontaneously with conservative management; however, large defects will need closure by primary closure using the adjacent mucosa across the socket to close the defect with a buccal fat pad advancement. This seal can be further augmented by the provision of a cover plate to the surgical site (and can be made when there is considered high risk of creating an OAC or for a planned surgical repair).

To prevent these situations from occurring, one must take great care to use gentle steady pressures when extracting teeth, avoiding excess forces or fast movements.

On other occasions, we might need to place things into the sinus. Dental implants are becoming increasingly popular. They are made predominantly of titanium, but treated in such a way that they osseointegrate with the bones of the jaw. This keeps them stable, prevents infection and allows them to withstand the forces that arise within the jaw. However, on occasion there is not enough bone for these implants to be placed, and in such cases, we are often asked to place bone grafts into the bottom of the sinus to create space. Once healed and established, this additional bone height allows implants to be placed and to osseointegrate. Sometimes, implants can even be placed into the bone of the zygoma, but such cases are usually reserved for situations when the amount of bone has been significantly reduced – for example, after a cancer resection.

7.6 SKIN CANCERS ON THE NOSE AND CHEEK

Skin cancers are managed in conjunction with dermatologists and oncologists as part of a skin-cancer multidisciplinary team (MDT). The central face is a high-risk site for the development of skin cancers such as basal cell carcinomas and squamous cell carcinomas. These cancers often require surgical excision. This can be done via Mohs micrographic surgery, where lesions are excised and microscopically assessed there and then to confirm that the tumours have been removed in their entirety before finishing the procedure. They can also be excised by a wide local excision, where the cancers are removed with a 4–6mm cuff of normal-looking skin tissue around the tumour before being sent to the lab. Although these numbers sound small, they lead to considerable defects in aesthetically sensitive areas. Coupled with the complex 3D shape of the nose, and to a lesser extent the cheek, reconstructing these defects once the cancers have been removed can be challenging – but also immensely satisfying.

We can close these defects primarily; sometimes we allow wounds to heal via secondary intention. Sometimes we use a scaffolding material to aid this process. Often, we prefer to use local skin flaps to help close these areas. Here, we use our knowledge of the relaxed skin tension lines to shift skin from areas that have more laxity to areas that have less movement, to allow us to close defects that we would otherwise not be able to.

Sometimes parts of the cartilaginous framework (alar cartilages) that support the nostrils also need to be removed. To reconstruct this area, we often use a conchal cartilage from the bowl of the ear to replace the alar cartilage, which gives the nostril its shape. Occasionally, for large defects, we need to perform a forehead flap, taking a flap of skin from the forehead and turning it around to rebuild the nose. After a few weeks, when it has gained a blood supply from the nasal area, the flap pedicle can be divided from the forehead region.

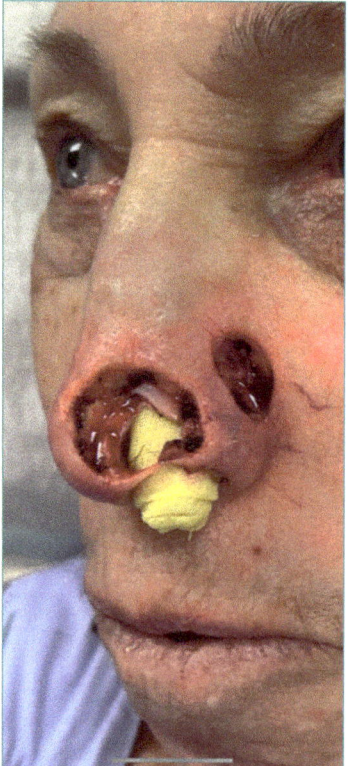

Figure 7.11a: Pre-op photo of defect post excision of skin cancer on left nasal tip and lateral nasal wall region. Picture courtesy of Mr. Richard Cobb

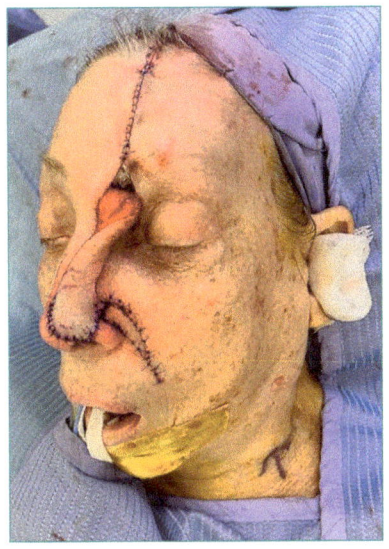

Figure 7.11b: Post-op after inset of forehead flap to address nasal tip defect and V-Y advancement flap of left cheek to the defect site. Picture courtesy of Mr. Richard Cobb

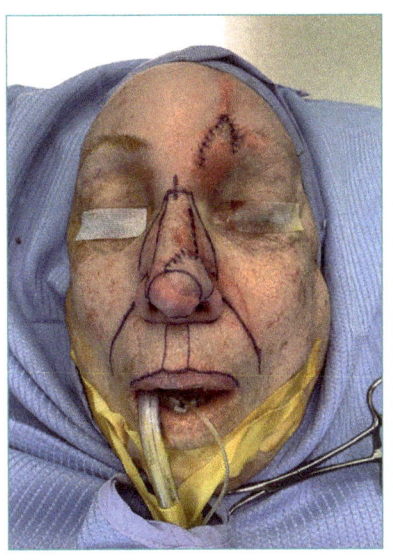

Figure 7.11c: Post-op after division of pedicled flap and closure at donor site. Picture courtesy of Mr. Richard Cobb

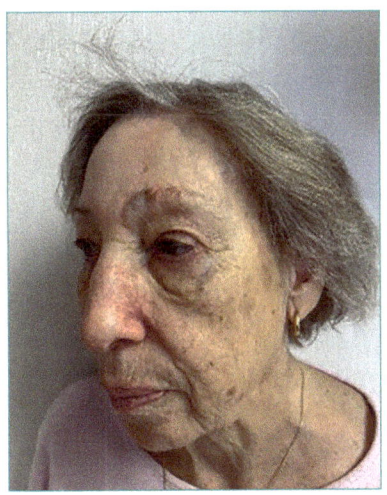

Figure 7.11d: Post-op at six months. Picture courtesy of Mr. Richard Cobb

Reviewing this chapter, you'll now appreciate that the midfacial third is a complex region involving the nose and upper jaw, along with the structures housed within the bones and the soft tissue superficial to them. This chapter has walked you through some of the important problems that patients present with in these regions, and introduced the principles that surgeons use to manage them.

CHAPTER 8: SKIN PATHOLOGY AND AESTHETIC SURGERY

8.1 SKIN CANCER

We briefly touched upon this in Chapter 6, where we just looked at cutaneous malignancy on the forehead. Let's now consider other presentations in other parts of the head and neck region.

8.1.1 MALIGNANT MELANOMA

Skin cancer is extremely common. Many of us will have a friend or relative with experience of some form of skin cancer, or personal experience of our own, so quite often these can be a talking point at social events. Skin cancers are generally divided into non-melanoma skin cancers (BCCs and SCCs) and malignant melanoma. While melanoma only represents 5% of skin cancers, it accounts for a significant majority of skin-cancer-related deaths. Sadly, despite public awareness and education, its incidence has doubled in the last 40 years.

Dentists get to observe patients close up and frequently have a regular review of patients, so you are well placed to advise patients about skin changes that you may notice as part of your regular review.

Risk Factors

Melanoma can develop in otherwise normal skin, or from pre-existing pigmented lesions. Like other forms of skin cancer, ultra-violet (UV) light exposure is considered the primary cause. However, unlike non-melanoma skin cancers, melanoma is perceived to be a consequence of intense sun exposure (burning is a key factor in particular).

The important risk factors to consider when taking a 'melanoma' history from anybody are as follows:

1. Pre-existing pigmented lesions
2. Age
3. Fair skin
4. Immunodeficiency
5. Family history.

Clinical Features

On examination, melanoma can have some classic clinical features. Pigmented lesions especially can be risk-assessed using an ABCDE approach.

- **A** – **A**symmetry
- **B** – Irregular **B**orders
- **C** – At least two different **C**olours in the lesion
- **D** – **D**iameter >6mm
- **E** – **E**levation of lesion

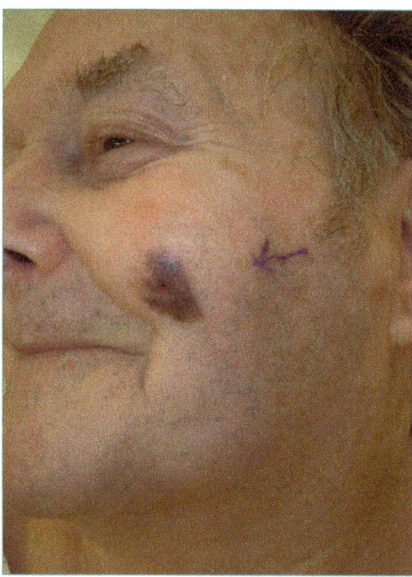

Figure 8.1: When assessing pigmented lesions, it is essential to use the ABCDE approach. Here, this suggested that the patient had a possible malignant melanoma. Picture courtesy of Mr. Stephen Walsh

Using this assessment system, you should be able to differentiate a potential melanoma from a common mole.

Management

When a melanoma is suspected, removal (excisional biopsy) is recommended, with a variable margin from 0.5cm to 2cm depending on stage and location. This provides a biopsy that represents the entire clinically visible lesion and therefore provides the best chance of an accurate diagnosis. (Importantly, an incisional or 'punch' biopsy, which only samples part of the lesion, might miss a crucially important area of deeper invasion.)

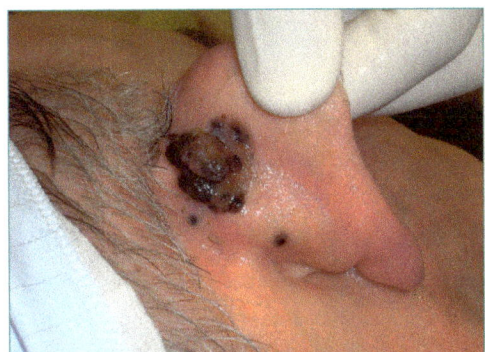

Figure 8.2: This gentleman presented with a pigmented lesion behind the right pinna. This was confirmed as malignant melanoma. Picture courtesy of Mr. Stephen Walsh

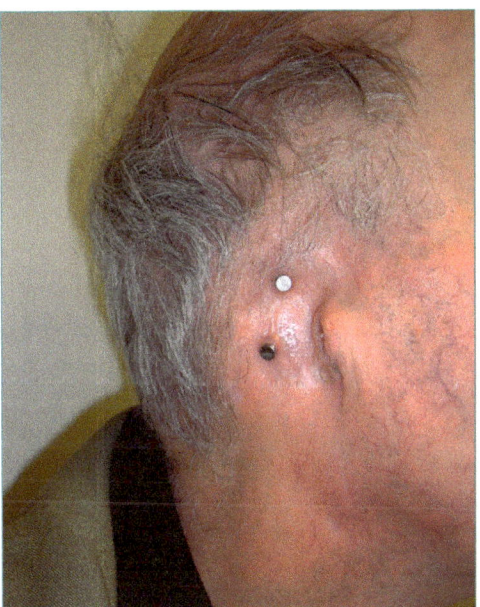

Figure 8.3: In order to potentially cure the patient, excisional biopsy meant pinnectomy, or removal of the ear. In order to provide reconstruction, titanium implants were placed into the temporal bone. Picture courtesy of Mr. Stephen Walsh

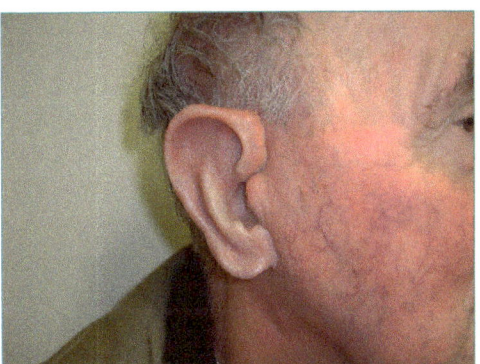

Figure 8.4: Once the implants had fully osseointegrated, a prosthesis was made by the laboratory which would be anchored onto the implants. Picture courtesy of Mr. Stephen Walsh

Staging

Today, it is established practice to measure the Breslow thickness. This is the thickness (in mm) measured from the granular layer of the epidermis to the deepest layer of identifiable tumour cells. Essentially, it measures how deep into the tissues the melanoma cells have growth. The greater the depth of growth, the worse the prognosis. This helps both stage the patient and provide a subsequent margin for further (definitive) wide local excision at a later date.

Melanoma has a tendency of metastasising to distant sites, so CT of the lungs, abdomen, pelvis and brain is often recommended by the MDT, where all these cases are discussed.

Sentinel Lymph Node Biopsy (SLNB)

Sentinel lymph node biopsy is widely considered to be the most accurate means of staging regional lymph nodes in melanoma. As we described in the Chapter 2 section on head and neck cancer, this is a staging procedure to check for regional spread – it is not a treatment. It involves the administration of a radioisotope tracer prior to nuclear imaging on the same day as surgery. Furthermore, blue dye is also injected into the site of the skin tumour. Using nuclear imaging and a specialised probe, the 'sentinel node' (the first draining node(s) from the anatomical region of the tumour) can be removed through a small neck incision and histologically checked for possible tumour cells. In this way, the stage of the tumour, from the point of view of regional spread, can be better assessed.

Treatment

Despite the advances in modern medicine, surgical excision of melanoma (at an early stage) is still the most effective treatment for malignant melanoma in terms of an attempt at complete cure. The excisional margin is determined by the Breslow thickness of the lesion. Melanoma management is always discussed at an MDT, with input from dermatologists, oncologists, pathologists, radiologists and surgeons (such as ENT, OMFS and plastics).

When there is regional-lymph-node disease in the head and neck, confirmed with ultrasound-guided fine-needle aspiration cytology (FNAC) or core biopsy, or by sentinel lymph node biopsy, a neck dissection with or without a superficial parotidectomy is performed, depending on the original location of the melanoma (for example, an anterior scalp or cheek melanoma can spread to the parotid gland nodes, hence it being included in the surgery).

Metastatic Disease

The presence of distant metastatic disease provides a poor prognosis. In these cases, sometimes the best course of treatment is 'palliation', to make the patient more comfortable, rather than aiming to cure the disease. This can be achieved through surgery, chemotherapy, immunotherapy and radiotherapy, or a combination of these. Treatment will always be discussed and agreed by the multidisciplinary team (MDT).

8.2 NON-MELANOMA SKIN CANCER (NMSC)

Non-melanoma cancers are the overwhelming majority of skin cancers arising in the head and neck – these are basal cell carcinomas (BCC), the commonest skin cancer, and squamous cell carcinomas (SCC). Fortunately, providing they are caught early, both are quite curable, though SCC does have a risk of metastasis to the regional lymph nodes. Nevertheless, it's important to remember that somebody who has had a skin cancer (regardless of complete cure) is at high risk of having similar cancers in the future and therefore requires a vigilant monitoring process for life. The key risk factors to consider when you suspect non-melanoma skin cancer are:

- Chronic exposure to UV light (burning is a concern but, unlike melanoma, it is the long-term history of UV exposure that is thought to be more relevant)
- Immunosuppression
- Genetic conditions
- Fair skin
- Premalignant conditions or lesions such as Bowen's disease (a scaly-like skin rash that histologically appears as carcinoma in situ) or actinic keratosis (also known as 'solar keratosis'; found typically in sun-bearing areas such as the forehead, scalp, ears, nose, cheeks and chin).

8.2.1 BASAL CELL CARCINOMA (BCC)

This is the commonest skin cancer and we see a lot of it, particularly in the southern parts of the UK where there is more sunshine. BCCs are usually slow growing and they do not metastasise, but their common name, 'rodent ulcer', confirms that they can be locally destructive. BCCs are commonly found on the face, typically on the forehead, nose, ears and cheeks, wherever there is sun exposure. In large lesions, we sometimes have to remove the nose or ear, and in cases of extreme neglect, even the orbital contents.

There are numerous clinical forms of BCC such as cystic, nodular, morphoeic and superficial BCC. But most importantly, these can be divided into low risk – nodular and superficial BCCs – and high risk – morphoeic/infiltrative, micronodular or baso-squamous.

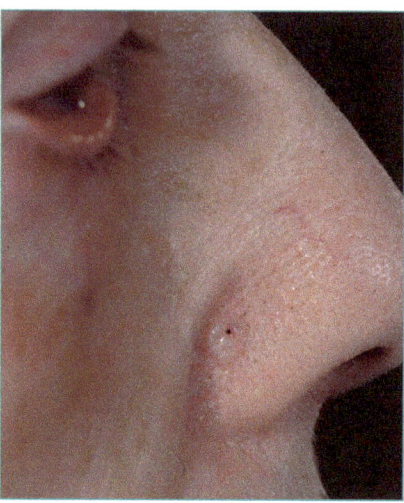

Figure 8.5: A classic BCC seen on the right nasal alar. Picture courtesy of Miss Nabeela Ahmed

8.2.2 SQUAMOUS CELL CARCINOMA (SCC)

Squamous cell carcinomas typically present as an indurated nodular lesion that may ulcerate, with a classically 'punched-out' appearance (unlike the more 'pearly rolled edge' of an ulcerating BCC); nevertheless, the two may often look similar clinically but differ histologically. These tumours can also present with a classic 'keratin horn', which is frequently mistaken by elderly patients and even healthcare professionals as dry 'crusty' skin. Other 'crusty' (flatter) patches of skin are more commonly actinic keratoses but even these have the potential to transform into an SCC. Like melanoma, SCC will be discussed at a skin MDT for best patient care. Another differential to consider here would be a keratoacanthoma.

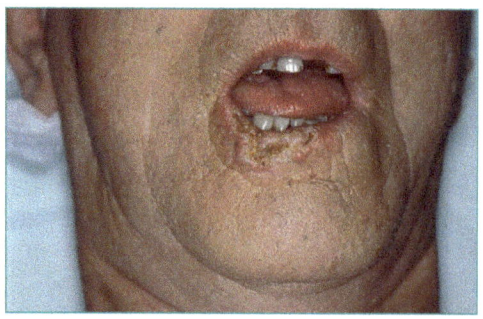

Figure 8.6: This gentleman presented with a crusting ulcer with 'rolled' edges. This was later confirmed as cutaneous SCC. Picture courtesy of Mr. Andrew Sidebottom

Diagnosis

Diagnosis of either form of non-melanoma skin cancer (NMSC) is usually achievable on clinical grounds alone. However, when in doubt, histological confirmation is achieved before definitive treatment, and this is achieved using either an incisional biopsy (of which punch biopsy is a type) or exfoliative cytology (skin scrapings – although this is relatively uncommon and not as diagnostically informative as a formal incisional biopsy).

Staging

If the patient presents with no evidence of cervical lymph node involvement, then there is no need for cross-sectional imaging. However, when nodal involvement is suspected, cross-sectional imaging of the neck and parotid should be performed and an FNA (or even better, a core biopsy) should be performed on clinically palpable enlarged nodes.

Treatment

BCC

Excision of the lesion is widely accepted as the gold standard. Depending upon the presence of high-risk features, the lesion is usually excised with a 4–5mm margin of normal tissue, which results in the clearance of disease in 95% of lesions. Exceptions are larger, infiltrative and morphoeic BCCs, which, by their nature, can make it difficult to establish surgical margins. As a result, wider margins are used to increase the chance of complete excision. Other management strategies are:

- Mohs micrographic surgery (step-by-step excision over several hours, using immediate frozen section histology to establish whether the tumour has been completely excised)
- Destructive techniques (e.g. curettage, cryosurgery or laser)
- Non-surgical
    - o Photodynamic therapy
    - o Immune modulators
- Radiotherapy.

SCC

Following MDT discussion, surgical excision is the treatment of choice, with a 95% clearance being achieved with a margin of 4mm for low-risk lesions, and a 6mm margin required for high-risk lesions. Other possible approaches include Mohs surgery, curettage and cautery or cryotherapy (the latter two used only by experienced practitioners). Radiotherapy is also an option.

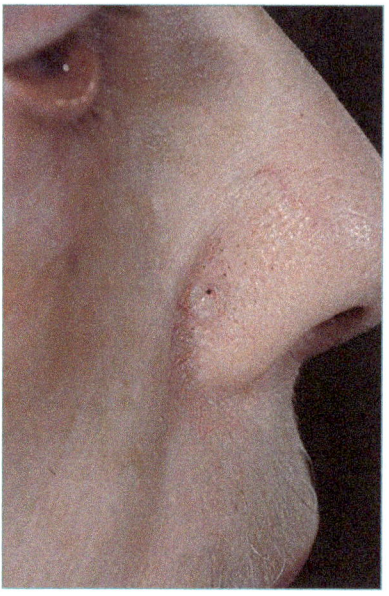

Figure 8.7: Lateral view of BCC on the lateral aspect of the nasal alar. Picture courtesy of Miss Nabeela Ahmed

Regional metastatic disease

This occurs in around 5% of cutaneous SCCs. If there is regional-lymph-node involvement and no evidence of distant metastatic spread (e.g. to the lungs) then surgery in the form of a neck dissection with or without a superficial parotidectomy (depending on the site of the tumour), because of the lymphatic drainage involving the parotid gland, may be the treatment with the best chance of cure, potentially alongside postoperative (adjuvant) radiotherapy.

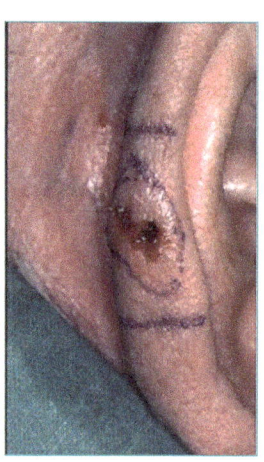

Figure 8.8: This patient presented with a lesion on the right pinna. Diagnosis can be challenging, as SCC can closely resemble BCC. In these instances, incisional biopsy can be useful. Picture courtesy of Professor P. Brennan

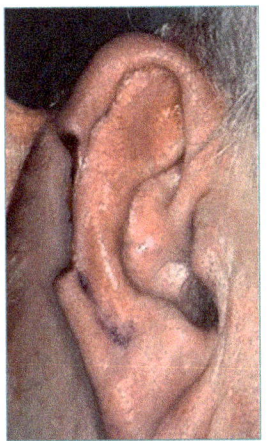

Figure 8.9: Excision of the lesion with a recommended margin can result in unsightly defects. Picture courtesy of Professor P. Brennan

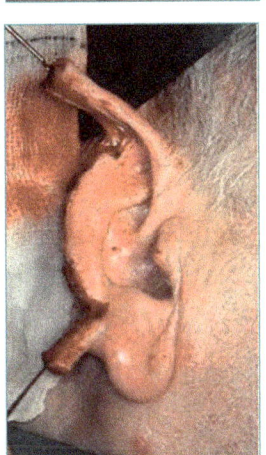

Figure 8.10: An OMF surgeon is also trained in reconstructive surgery. Such techniques were employed here. Picture courtesy of Professor P. Brennan

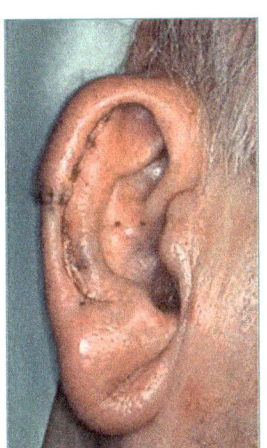

Figure 8.11: The final result! Picture courtesy of Professor P. Brennan

8.3 BENIGN SKIN TUMOURS

8.3.1 KERATOACANTHOMA

Keratoacanthomas mimic cutaneous squamous cell carcinomas in appearance, but most notably, these regress with time. Despite this, their diagnosis can be incredibly challenging clinically. As such, histological assessment is in the patient's best interest and they are generally treated by excision.

8.3.2 LIPOMA

A lipoma is a benign fat tumour that can occur in the subcutaneous tissues as well as elsewhere in the body, including the gut and within skeletal muscle, for example. They can even be found in the mouth. They are completely harmless and slow growing. Most notably, on examination they will feel dough-like and mobile within the skin and/or under the mucosa in the lip or cheek. Quite often the patient will report that it has been there for many years and has slowly grown over that time. Treatment is by simple excision. Sometimes an ultrasound can be useful to give an idea of size or proximity to surrounding structures.

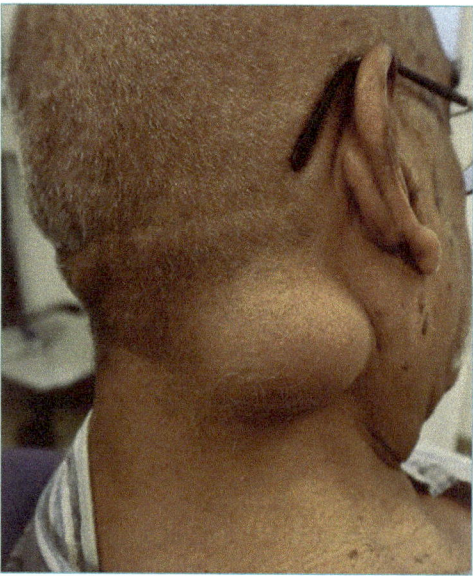

Figure 8.12: This gentleman presented with a slow-growing, soft lump in the posterior neck. Ultrasound was highly suggestive of a lipoma. Picture courtesy of Mr. Madan Ethunandan

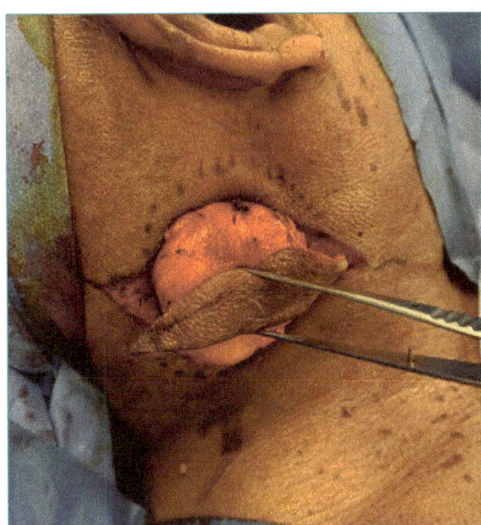

Figure 8.13: The lump was removed. As these are slow-growing, benign masses, they often act as skin expanders. Upon removal, any excess or redundant skin should also be excised. Picture courtesy of Mr. Madan Ethunandan

8.4 AESTHETIC SKIN SURGERY

Humans are social animals. Our faces are complex structures that play an important role in how we engage through social interaction. How we perceive the way we look also has impacts on our own psychology and can affect us in profound ways. While many of the problems you have read about in this book look to manage and correct functional problems – a bleeding nose, a fractured jaw or a growing tumour – it is not unusual to meet patients who don't have functional problems. Instead, they are not happy with the appearance of their face, whether that be due to a previous injury, a product of ageing or simply something about their facial appearance that they feel to be unappealing.

Facial aesthetics is a broad field and perhaps one where the craft and judgment of an oral and maxillofacial or plastic surgeon are particularly highlighted. Aesthetics can be impacted in a number of ways and at a number of levels. Sometimes they are limited to the cutaneous layer. For example, patients may be concerned about how scars from previous operations have healed. As you have read, we often work hard to hide facial scars in areas of the face that naturally heal well, but sometimes, particularly in traumatic injuries, this is not possible. This can leave often quite conspicuous scars in aesthetically sensitive areas. Sometimes, the subcutaneous tissues and fat beneath the skin can be affected, leading to asymmetry or the appearance of swellings or depressions. Muscle weakness or atrophy, either through direct injury, ageing or disrupted nerve supply, can compromise aesthetics, as can any change in the underlying bony or cartilaginous contour.

Regardless, our knowledge of facial anatomy and physiology becomes very useful as we try to address these patients' concerns: what is it exactly that is concerning the patient and what are the specific underlying causes of the aesthetic problems? The key tenets of any medical assessment remain fundamental: a thorough history and examination, carefully unpicking the key concerns and worries, are vital. Then, importantly, once these have been explored, we consider how best to correct the issue. There are highly varied options either to correct the underlying problems or to mask them in a way that no longer appears unaesthetic. The most straightforward way to think of these is as non-surgical or surgical treatments.

Non-surgical treatments are things like botulinum toxin injections, dermal fillers or resurfacing procedures. Botulinum toxin type A (or 'Botox', which is actually a brand name) works by disrupting the transmission of impulses at the neuromuscular junction and thus, when carefully injected into specific sites, can serve to decrease the dynamic skin creases by paralysing some of the muscles of facial expression and reducing dynamic wrinkling. Common areas that are injected are the frown lines over the nasal bridge and forehead, and the crow's feet over the lateral aspects of the orbits.

Dermal fillers are injectable substances that are used to fill out the deep grooves around the face and smooth out problematic wrinkles. Resurfacing techniques tend to involve removal of the very superficial layers of problematic areas, and allowing the new formation of healthier tissue.

There tends to be lots of overlap between different surgical options, but they can largely be thought of as '-*plasties*', 'lifts' and 'grafts or implants'.

'*Plasties*' are a group of terms that highlight how a surgeon alters the appearance of a particular area. For example, a blepharoplasty modifies the appearance of the upper or lower eyelids; a rhinoplasty reshapes the nose; an otoplasty can alter the shape of the ear; while a genioplasty changes the shape or size of the chin. These often involve alterations in different elements of these structures such as skin, underlying fat or bone. Importantly, there are nuances and complexities involved with each of them and huge variation in how they are performed from surgeon to surgeon. Many of these techniques can be used to manage patients wanting facial-feature feminisation, and are increasingly practised by surgeons. In addition, some of the skills can be used to augment the facial profile and can be done with soft-tissue-work alone, alongside including the use of custom-made implants (for example, to help recontour the lower border of the mandible). This is a growing area of management in an aesthetically aware population group.

Whether secondary to an ageing face or due to traumatic muscle or nerve injuries, over time the tissues of the face can begin to sag, droop or wrinkle due to the loss of underlying muscle tone. In these situations, various different *lifting* procedures may benefit patients. The wrinkles in the forehead or eyebrow can be addressed using brow lifts. These can be done either directly, with an incision in the forehead itself (hidden in the creases or the hairlines), or using endoscopic techniques which use several small, inconspicuous incisions instead. In both cases, the skin, fat and muscles are pulled up, stretched and anchored to give a rejuvenated appearance. Other lifting procedures include the rhytidectomy – or facelift – where again, the surgeon's knowledge of facial anatomy (for example, the same anatomy encountered when performing parotid-gland surgery) becomes vital. In these procedures, we make use of the SMAS layer (the superficial musculo-aponeurotic system) that serves to interconnect many of the intricate muscles of facial expression. We know that it is the muscle action of the face that leads to wrinkles, so simply stretching the skin is perhaps not the best way to rejuvenate the face. However, we can make a hidden skin incision and raise a facial skin flap then, importantly (and with care, because the facial nerve lies just deep to this layer), we can dissect the SMAS layer, lift it and remove any excess and re-anchor it – thus stretching out the muscle layer. We can then drape the skin over this, which is a far more effective way to reduce wrinkling and rejuvenate the patient's facial appearance.

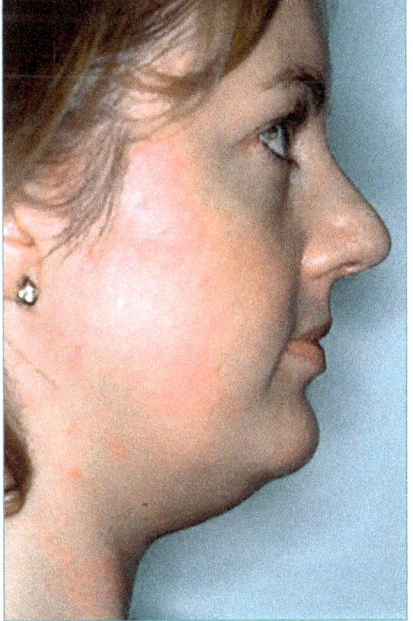

Figure 8.14: This patient presented with concerns of an ageing face. Picture courtesy of Mr. Andrew Sidebottom

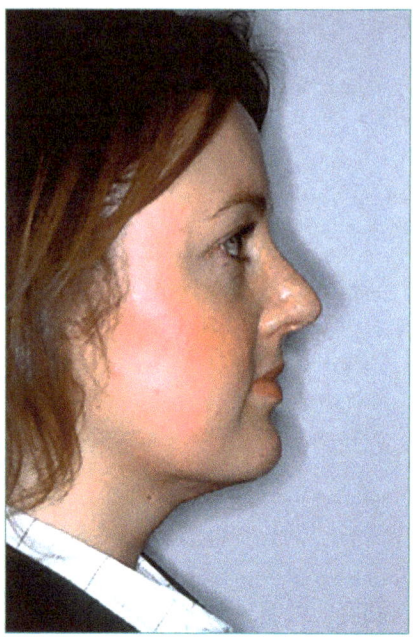

Figure 8.15: She underwent a neck lift and submental lipectomy. This resulted in a more youthful appearance. Picture courtesy of Mr. Andrew Sidebottom

In some situations, stretching or reshaping what is already there is perhaps not appropriate, and an area may need further augmentation. Similar to dermal fillers, autogenous (i.e. the patient's own) fat can be harvested – for example, from the abdomen, groin or thigh. This can either be a block of dermal fat which can be placed en-bloc in the recipient site or a liquefied form of fat transfer: lipo-suctioned fat is centrifuged and then reinjected to a particular region to bulk out a contracted scar, or to fill a defect caused by an untreated frontal bone fracture, for example. Other defects, particular those caused by underlying bony defects, can be masked with synthetic graft material, bone grafts or cartilage. Of course, many of these techniques are used alongside each other, and choosing which work well together can take many years to fully appreciate!

CHAPTER 9: ORAL AND MAXILLOFACIAL SURGERY – CAREER AND RESEARCH OPPORTUNITIES

9.1 BACKGROUND

Arguably, in no other speciality are you exposed to, and trained in, the plethora of soft- and hard-tissue skills, across both paediatric and adult patients, with both benign and malignant disease, as you've seen showcased in this book on OMFS.

Historically, OMFS was a dental speciality born from the necessity for dentists and oral surgeons to enter the hospital setting to treat facial trauma. As of 1995, all OMFS consultants required dual qualification. The 2008 Postgraduate Medical Education and Training Board (PMETB) review provided further evidence for the requirement of both medical and dental qualifications. So, OMFS is now one of the 10 UK surgical specialities and as such is regulated by the General Medical Council (GMC).

Despite being a medical speciality, OMFS teaching in the medical undergraduate curriculum has been slow (hence the requirement for the medical version of this book). While the OMFS workforce was almost exclusively made up of 'dental-first' surgeons who completed a medical degree after working as an OMFS junior, over the past 10–15 years there has been a changing tide, with around half of newly appointed OMFS speciality registrars (StRs) now being 'medicine-first' trainees. This reflects the fact that of the relatively few undergraduate and postgraduate medics in the UK who gain exposure to OMFS, a significant proportion love it so much that they will go on to get a second degree in dentistry and become an oral and maxillofacial surgeon. This harmonious balance of trainee backgrounds between 'medicine first' and 'dentistry first' creates a rich and diverse speciality workforce.

After browsing through the rest of this book, we hope you will have come to realise that OMFS is a diverse and interesting speciality. Despite being perceived as a 'niche' and unique speciality (given the need for dual qualification in both dentistry and medicine), it actually encompasses a huge range of conditions and surgical treatments that merge and are complemented by colleagues with ENT, plastic surgery, trauma, ophthalmology, neurosurgery, orthodontic and medical expertise.

Surgery can include cleft, craniofacial, orthognathic and dentoalveolar surgery, as well as skin, salivary gland, major head and neck cancer and free-flap reconstructions, plating facial fractures or exploring a patient's neck after penetrating neck trauma. As such, it straddles the divide between dentistry and medicine and is the primary referral source for dentists and from GPs for all problems of the face, mouth, neck and jaws. As we've seen in this book, OMFS sub-specialities include:

- Oral surgery
- Head and neck oncology and reconstruction
- Salivary-gland surgery
- Paediatric OMFS
- Craniofacial and orthognathic surgery
- TMJ
- Cleft
- Facial aesthetics
- Craniofacial trauma (including both the primary and secondary management).

9.2 BRITISH ASSOCIATION OF ORAL AND MAXILLOFACIAL SURGEONS (BAOMS)

BAOMS hosts an annual scientific meeting/conference which is a superb way of maintaining contact with the speciality and being afforded opportunities to present work in the form of posters and verbal presentations (all of which are requirements for progress and often graded and used to shortlist for entry to training and grants, etc.).

The BAOMS also supports a Junior Trainee Group (JTG) and a Fellows in Training group. They have regular meetings across the year and representatives in most medical and dental schools, as well as regional representatives to help network and support peers aspiring to be OMFS surgeons. They provide a great deal of informal advice and support. More details are available via the BAOMS website. The JTG function primarily as an online community via a well-established online-based group which provides peer support and advice.

9.3 CAREER PATHWAYS

What often confuses dental students or trainees interested in OMFS as a career is the training pathway – in other words, when to do the second degree. You can apply as soon as you finish dentistry, but financially you need to consider the cost impact of this prompt return (as you will be very unlikely to be placed on a shortened course). Many of you will undertake dental core-training hospital posts and/or foundation dental training and complete the MFDS exam. The decision of where to be based often comes down to exposure to OMFS during dental school and foundation and/or dental core-training location, in addition to local opportunities.

It is a huge undertaking to return to complete a second degree, and you should try and gain a wide breadth of experience in OMFS, ideally in an OMFS dental core-training post. If nothing else, this is so as to be able to support yourself with work as a student and to maintain your contact with the speciality whilst on the second degree.

The nature of recruitment to OMFS and the availability of second-degree places, especially those shortened courses for dentally qualified individuals, change regularly, so please review up-to-date information regarding this on the BAOMS Junior Trainee Group's webpage (https://jtgonline.org/).

Up-to-date information on the OMFS training pathways can also be found on the BAOMS website at:
https://www.baoms.org.uk/professionals/careers_in_omfs.aspx.

On a yearly basis, BAOMS will advertise and support workshops delivered to support those thinking of and embarking upon the second-degree process. For further information, look at:
https://www.baoms.org.uk/professionals/baoms_second_degree_workshops.aspx.

9.4 RESEARCH

Despite the potential for a slightly longer training pathway, some OMFS trainees still endeavour to undertake higher degrees to follow an academic surgical career. With the plethora of potential sub-specialities listed above, the scope for research is vast. Because of the historic roots in dentistry, much of the academic work was previously undertaken within dental schools alone. However, with the many advances in the scope of surgery performed (including complex head and neck and craniomaxillofacial procedures), OMFS was formally recognised as a surgical speciality within medicine rather than dentistry in 1994, and now the academic base of OMFS has expanded into medical schools and allied groups – for example, genomics research.

OMFS has a particularly strong reputation for research into head and neck cancer and reconstruction – leading on national and international clinical trials, and with several units within the UK undertaking important basic science and translational research.

The academic pathway in OMFS is not dissimilar to those of other surgical specialities, with options to complete academic clinical fellowships (ACF) and academic clinical lectureships (ACL) during both medical and dental training. However, you don't need a higher degree to get involved in OMFS research: from student to registrar, there are abundant opportunities to undertake potentially high-impact research and get some decent publications to your name. Oral and maxillofacial surgeons recognise the importance of furthering their speciality and, having completed two degrees, are optimally placed to do so.

If you are interested in research then go to the BAOMS website (www.baoms.org.uk) and check out the Maxillofacial Trainee Research Collaborative (MTReC – https://www.maxfaxtrainee.co.uk/), in addition to the UK Society of Oral and Maxillofacial Academic Surgeons' website (https://abaoms.org).

Hopefully, we have through this book provided you with an array of knowledge and clinical cases, and showcased the breadth of our speciality. Please do let us know if you wish we had covered additional topics.

INDEX

Actinic keratosis   131, 132
Alveolar bone graft   39, 40
Ameloblastoma   64, 68
Anaplastic carcinoma   99
Anastomosis   30, 31, 33, 82
Angular cheilitis   22
Anterior open bite   4, 49
Anterolateral thigh flap   30
Apicectomy   37, 65
Arteriovenous malformation   94, 95
Arthrocentesis   60
Arthroscopy   60
Atypical facial pain   79
Basal cell carcinoma (BCC)   110, 123, 127, 131–2, 133, 134
Bell's palsy   80
Bilateral sagittal split osteotomy   57
Bimaxillary osteotomy   57
Black hairy tongue   22
Blepharoplasty   138
Blood tests   7, 10–11, 79, 98, 99
Bony exostoses (tori)   6, 27
Botulinum toxin type   138
Bowen's disease   131
Branchial arches   94
Branchial cyst   94
Breslow thickness   130
Burning mouth syndrome   79
Candidiasis   20–1
Canines   3, 36–7
Carcinoma in situ   18, 131
Cellulitis   90
Cerebrospinal fluid   104
Cervical lymphadenopathy   6, 73, 89, 91
Cervical sinus   94
Chronic hyperplastic candidiasis   20
Cleft lip   38–41, 43, 119
Cleft palate   38–41, 43, 54, 119
Conchal cartilage   124
Cranial nerves   7, 78, 101
Craniosynostosis   109
Cricothyroidotomy   12

Crow's feet   138
CT scan   8, 9, 45, 59, 64, 67, 70, 104, 106
Dental caries   3, 8, 34
Dental implants   9, 33, 34, 37–8, 123
Dental sinus   25, 89
Dental trauma   12, 41
Dentoalveolar surgery   34–8, 142
Denture-induced hyperplasia   25
Dermal fillers   138, 140
Dermoid cyst   91
DiGeorge syndrome   39
Dislocation   62
Distraction osteogenesis   40, 58, 110
EBV (Epstein Barr Virus)   22, 28, 91
Enophthalmos   107
Epidermoid cyst   91
Epistaxis   49, 119
Erythema multiforme   17–18
Erythroplakia   18, 22
Excisional biopsy   7, 25, 128, 129
Exodontia   34
Extra-capsular dissection   75
Face lift   82, 139
Facial nerve   43, 48, 60, 71–5, 81, 82, 84–6, 97, 102, 103, 139
Facial palsy   80–2
Facial reanimation   82
Fascial layers   74, 90
Fat transfer   140
Fibroepithelial polyp   25–6
Fibula   30, 33, 34, 37
Fine-needle aspiration cytology (FNAC)   73, 89, 92, 94, 96, 98, 130
Follicular carcinoma   98–9
Foramen caecum   92
Fordyce spots   21
Forehead flap   102, 124, 125
Frey's syndrome   75, 77
Frontal bone   2, 3, 51, 101, 104–5, 140
Frontal sinus   101, 104
Fronto-nasal duct   101
Fronto-nasal prominence   43

Genioplasty 57, 58, 138
Geographic tongue 21
Guillain-Barré 80
Hairy oral leukoplakia 22
Hemithyroidectomy 98
Herpes zoster 80
HIV 22, 91
House–Brackmann scale 80, 97
Human papilloma virus (HPV) 28
Hypoglobus 107–8
Impaction 34–7
Incisional biopsy 19, 20, 28, 128, 133, 134
Joint replacement 64
Keratin horn 132
Keratoacanthoma 132, 136
Keratocystic odontogenic tumour (KCOT) 64, 66, 68
Keratosis 18, 19, 21, 131
Laceration 2, 12, 81, 83–4, 86
Lateral canthotomy 12
Le Fort fractures 4, 48–50, 57
Leukoedema 21
Leukoplakia 18, 19, 22
Lichen planus 19–20
Lichenoid reaction 20
Lipoma 136–7
Ludwig's angina 90–1
Lymph node 7, 16, 28, 29, 30, 73–4, 89, 94, 95–6, 130, 131, 133, 134
Lymphoma 95
Malignant melanoma 7, 127–31
Median rhomboid glossitis 22
Medication relation osteonecrosis of the jaws (MRONJ) 68–9
Medullary carcinoma 99
Minor salivary glands 25, 71, 77
Mohs micrographic surgery 123, 133
Monson's classification 86
MRI 29, 59, 73, 79, 94, 95, 98
Mucocele 25–6, 77
Mucosal melanoma 22–3
Nasal packing 120–1
Nasal splint 118
Naso-orbito-ethmoidal fractures 50, 116
Nasolacrimal duct 115
Neck dissection 24, 29–30, 98–9, 130, 134

Neck lumps 7, 28, 88–9, 97, 99
Obstructive sleep apnoea 53
Occipitomental radiographs 9, 53
Occlusal radiograph 76
Oculo-cardiac reflex 108
Odontogenic Keratocyst 64, 66
Operculum 35
OPG 8, 33, 35, 37, 45, 59, 61, 63, 64, 65, 67, 68, 122
Ophthalmoplegia 108
Oral cancer 15, 16, 24, 28–33
Oral submucous fibrosis 18, 28
Orbital compartment syndrome 108–9
Oroantral communication 122–3
Orthognathic surgery 4, 39, 40, 53–4, 57, 142
Osteoradionecrosis (ORN) 69–70
Osteotomy 57
Otoplasty 138
PA mandible 8, 45, 61
Papillary carcinoma 98, 99
Paramedian forehead flap 102, 124, 125
Paranasal sinuses 115
Parathyroid tumours 99
Pemphigoid 6, 17
Pemphigus 5, 17
Penetrating neck injuries 86–8, 142
Peri-tonsillar abscess 89
Pericoronitis 35
Photodynamic therapy 133
Pinnectomy 129
Pleomorphic adenoma 73, 75
Post-herpetic neuralgia 80
Proptosis 108–9
Punch biopsy 128, 133
Radial forearm free flap 30–2
Radiotherapy 29, 69–70, 74, 110, 131, 133, 134
Ramsay Hunt syndrome 80, 81
Ranula 25–7, 77
Reactive lymph node 96
Recurrent aphthous stomatitis 17
Relaxed skin tension lines 111, 112, 124
Retrobulbar haemorrhage 12, 108, 109
Rhinoplasty 39, 41, 57, 58, 118, 138
Rhytidectomy 139
Salivary glands 24, 25, 70, 71–7, 142
Sebaceous cyst 91
Sentinel lymph node biopsy 29, 130

Septoplasty   118
Shingles   80
Sialogram   75
Sialolithiasis   75
Sinusitis   78, 122
Sistrunk procedure   93, 94
SMAS   74, 139
Solar keratosis   131
Space-occupying lesion   79
Speech and language therapy   39, 110
Squamous cell carcinoma (SCC)   16, 24–5, 28, 29, 30, 32, 110, 123, 127, 131, 132–5, 136
Staging   28–9, 130, 133
Static reanimation   82
Stickler syndrome   39
Stridor   98
Superficial parotidectomy   71, 75, 130, 134
Synovial fluid   58
Telecanthus   116
Temporomandibular joint   2, 3, 8, 43, 58–64, 78
Temporomandibular joint dysfunction   59–60, 62, 78
Tetanus   83–4
Third molar surgery   35
Thyroglossal cysts   92–4, 97, 99
Thyroid gland   25, 68, 92, 98, 99
Thyroidectomy   98–9
TNM system   29, 74
Tori/torus   6, 27
Tracheostomy   12, 30, 87, 88
Trauma zones   86–7
Trigeminal neuralgia   78–9
Ulcers   6, 11, 14–18, 24, 81, 131, 132
Ultrasound   28, 39, 73, 75, 89, 92, 94–5, 130, 136
Van der Woude syndrome   39
Varicella-zoster virus   80
Vascular malformation   94–5
Velopharyngeal insufficiency   40
White-eye orbital-floor fracture   108
Wisdom teeth (third molars)   3, 9, 35, 65, 119

www.ingramcontent.com/pod-product-compliance
Lightning Source LLC
LaVergne TN
LVHW072021060526
838200LV00008B/222